Writing My Way Through Cancer

Myra Schneider

Jessica Kingsley Publishers
London and Philadelphia

First published in the United Kingdom in 2003
by Jessica Kingsley Publishers
116 Pentonville Road
London N1 9JB, England
and
400 Market Street, Suite 400
Philadelphia, PA 19106, USA
www.jkp.com

Copyright © Myra Schneider 2003
Second impression 2004

Library of Congress Cataloging in Publication Data
Schneider, Myra, 1936-
    Writing my way through cancer / Myra Schneider.
        p. cm.
    Includes bibliographical references and index.
    ISBN 1-84310-113-0 (pbk. : alk. paper)
        1. Schneider, Myra, 1936--Health. 2. Breast--Cancer--Patients--United
States--Biography. 3. Creative writing--Therapeutic use. 4. Cancer patients' writings. I.
Title.

RC280.B8 S347 2003
362.1'9699449'0092--dc21
[B]   2002038909

British Library Cataloguing in Publication Data
A CIP catalogue record for this book is available from the British Library

ISBN 1 84310 113 0

Printed and Bound in Great Britain by
Athenaeum Press, Gateshead, Tyne and Wear

Contents

Part I: Journal

Part II: Writing Ideas

Poems in the book

Notes and Lists

*Half the royalties from this book are being donated
to the Helen Rollason Cancer Care Centre Appeal.*

A division of HEAL Cancer Charity, Reg. Charity No. 1052861

Acknowledgements

The author and Jessica Kingsley Publishers would like to express their thanks to the following authors and publishers for permission to reprint material:

Bloodaxe and Carole Satyamurti for 'Difficult Passages', 'Choosing the Furniture', 'I Shall Paint My Nails Red' from her sequence *Changing The Subject* in her *Selected Poems* (Bloodaxe 2000; Oxford University Press 1998).

Gill & Macmillan and Sheila Dainow, Vicki Golding and Jo Wright for two extracts by Vicki Golding and one by Jo Wright from *44½ Choices you can make if you have cancer* (Gill & Macmillan 2001).

Grevel Lindop for an extract from a letter.

Les Murray for extracts from correspondence.

Mary MacRae for an extract from her sonnet sequence: *Knitting* and her poem 'Appointment', also for permission to quote from her notebook.

Alicia Stubbersfield for her poem 'Goodbye to my left breast' and permission to use three extracts from her notebook.

Poems in this book have also appeared in the following magazines:

Poems by Mary MacRae in *Magma*, *Scintilla*.

Poems by Myra Schneider in *Magma*, *The North*, *Poetry London*, *Prop*, *Quadrant* (Australia), *Scintilla*

I should like to thank Erwin, my husband, for all the support he has given me both during the time of my illness and in preparing this book for publication. I should like to thank Mary MacRae for her sympathetic interest in the book and for commenting on it at every stage, also John Killick and Caroline Price for reading the text and offering insightful suggestions. I am grateful to Lynne Wycherley for checking the final script.

I also want to thank Sheila and Cyril Dainow for all their hospitality and kindness while I was ill.

As well as the people mentioned in the journal I should like to thank all the other friends who supported me during my illness and in particular: Nadine Brummer, Caroline Canale, Tricia Corob, Sheila Conroy – my sister, Martyn Crucefix, Phyllis and Max Glasman, Lucy Hamilton, Jenny and Den Harrington, Miriam Hastings, Liz Houghton, Myra Houlding, Nora Kingbourn, Nina Lazarus, Shirley and Paul Millichip, Hubert Moore, Pam Patel, Beryl Sabel, Pam and Wally Scott, Hylda Sims, Margaret Sutton, Isobel Thrilling, Doreen and Bill Wainwright, Frances Wilson, Joy Winterbottom, Grazyna Wloch.

Note

Occasionally the identity of an individual who appears in the journal has been disguised.

PART I

Journal

CHAPTER ONE

Investigation

12th January 2000

This morning I woke up relaxed in the cocoon of my bed and hugged the warmth in my woolly socks. Loving the normality of the sounds inside and outside the house, I blanked everything else out and listened to Erwin, my husband, opening a door. Then I heard a low rhythmic rumble gathering to the clatter of a train passing over the viaduct with its little rectangles of light. There was a grumble as it died away, the clanking calls of two or three geese flying over the park and the creak of the central heating. I didn't feel like surfacing from my muzziness but after a while I made myself look at the curtains and estimate from the light edging in what the time was. The brightness told me it wasn't early. Grudgingly I reached from my lair to check the time on my watch. It was much later than I'd guessed. I bounded out of bed and as I dressed I tuned in to what I'd be writing this morning. This was not only what I wanted to do today – today and every day for the last week – it was also a way of holding fear at bay.

It was last Wednesday that I discovered I'd been picked out – hounded out it felt like – and called back to the hospital. Each time I'd been for a routine mammogram in the Portakabin at the edge of the car park in the North Middlesex Hospital I'd not allowed myself to dwell on any possibilities, simply thought of it as a safety procedure to get out of the way and then forget. The letter I received last week was brief and smoothed things over by stating there was nothing to worry about at this stage – but how could I *not* worry? I was dizzy with apprehension that something had been found which would dismantle my life. A sword hung over me. I kept seeing its glitter of danger.

At the hospital the next day I was told, coldly it seemed to me, that there was a shadow on the ultrasound scan and asked if there was cancer in the family. The shadow was pointed out to me. Erwin saw it but I was too shaken to make out anything except a series of meaningless blurs. In any case I don't suppose I wanted to see. The breast cancer nurse, a solid woman with a youngish, generous face, stepped in at this point to explain in a friendly way that they needed to do a biopsy – to take a sample from the area in question. I was given a local anaesthetic. Even so the jab of the syringe was quite painful and I felt it as an attack on my poor, unoffending left breast.

The consultant radiologist wasn't abrasive but he didn't have a reassuring manner either. He also seemed to have difficulty in locating the spot from which he wanted to take a sample. More nurses gathered around. Why? Was there something specially noteworthy? My alarm grew. I tried to distract myself by looking at the readings on the computer screen. I didn't understand them but I was impressed that there was so much technical equipment to assist in diagnosing and treating illness now. I told myself I was lucky, that a few years ago this test was probably done under general anaesthetic.

Going home was awful. I'd nourished a hope that the sword above my head would be removed, the shadow pronounced a mistake or something very unimportant. Instead nothing had been resolved, my fear had been raised higher and I had no option but to live with it for four days while I waited for the result – a result which just might be that I had cancer. I was angry that my breast was wounded, that the dressing on it had to be kept dry so that I couldn't even have a proper bath.

I willed myself over the following days to get on with the long narrative poem I'd started the previous summer. Writing, total involvement in what I'm producing, has always been a way for me to cut out tension. Teaching or losing myself in a film or play also lifts me right out of myself.

To go to the hospital I had had to cancel the whole of my weekly session teaching communication and literacy to severely disabled adults at Flightways Day Centre. In the morning I managed to concentrate on developing material for a new section of the narrative poem and this helped me to keep my anxiety at a remove. After we'd parked the car we trudged some distance past great, grey, ungainly buildings without finding Out-Patients and I was soon in a panic. I spoke to a hospital worker who sent us back the way we'd come – we had managed to miss the Out-Patients' block even though it was beside the car park! Once inside the building I rushed down the corridor on the verge of tears in case we were late which, of course, we weren't. The clinic hadn't even started – I felt a complete fool.

A clerk working at an open desk in the dismal semi-basement hall was uninterested in our arrival and simply told us to sit down. I looked at the rows of mainly empty chairs. An elderly black woman was sitting alone, face blank, whole body passive as if resigned to a life of waiting. A woman, Italian I guessed, came in. Taut and queenly, she walked slowly followed by four unsmiling adult daughters in long dark coats and trendy boots. It could have been a ritual drama. They sat in complete silence and I had the sense that nothing ever happened here, that if people were sent to it they stagnated for ever. Hopelessness settled on me like ash.

After what seemed like a long time though I suspect it was no more than a quarter of an hour I saw, to my surprise and relief, the consultant radiologist and breast cancer nurse making their way down the long corridor. The nurse was carrying a huge wodge of files and I knew one of them must contain the verdict on me. The Italian lady was seen first. She was soon out and I was called in. It was a terrible anti-climax – the verdict wasn't a verdict: 'Although the results are negative we're not convinced we've taken a proper sample,' the radiologist explained.

'We'll do the test again, this time under X-ray to make sure we find the right spot. It's difficult to be accurate when the area is so small.'

In the nightmare I held onto this smallness. If I had a problem it could be dealt with – and I understood this as easily dealt with. It was depressing to find that the test could not be done again immediately as a fortnight was needed for my breast to heal. I asked if it was possible to avoid a Monday as it meant losing my weekly session teaching disabled adults.' Smiling, the radiologist said: 'Come in on the Thursday instead...'

I dread undergoing the test again and it will be worse sitting squashed against the X-ray machine. Worse still, I won't have any certainty for three weeks. I'm clinging to the minuteness of that 'shadow', keep telling myself that if there is something malign it will only need very minor treatment, that there may be no problem at all.

28th January

I've adjusted; there's no choice but to adjust. I've spoken to friends about my anxiety and they've been comforting: shadows often turn out to be nothing; most tumours are benign. The fig purple bruise on my breast has slowly faded. Until yesterday I've managed during the daytime, sometimes with a struggle, to sit on the fear I'm carrying. Ordinary life has been busy and immersing myself in it has been a way of making myself believe that it will continue. In the last two weeks I've given two poetry readings; one with eighty-year-old poet Elizabeth Bewick in Southampton. I've also given a tutorial, run my regular writing workshops and taught at Flightways each Monday.

At night it's been much harder. Terror breaks out, wraps itself round me, kicks sleep away. I've told myself many other people are living with fear so I must too. I've asked myself what people do with all this suffering, how it is voiced. I've taken sleeping pills but they haven't always worked and when they have my sleep has been turbulent. One night I dreamt a man who looked quite civilized was raping me. I struggled and struggled against the terror, trying to negotiate with him. In the end he seemed to agree I could keep my vest and pants on. When he climaxed I realized with relief that he had not been inside me. As soon as I woke up it struck me that the man had looked rather like a doctor friend I've lost touch with – someone who is, in fact, a very gentle person. Immediately I connected the dream with the biopsy, the attack on my breast.

Yesterday began very badly. We had to be at the hospital quite early for the biopsy and before breakfast I took the letter about the appointment out of a drawer to put in my bag. Glancing at it I saw the date I'd been given was *last* Thursday. It hadn't occurred to me that I'd be given an appointment earlier than the Monday first offered. Evidently I hadn't read the letter properly. I was appalled. My mistake meant I'd already put things back one week. If I wasn't fitted into this morning's clinic the delay would be even greater. Luckily Erwin is much less easily shaken than me and although I was urging him to phone up, he insisted the best thing to do was to arrive early before the clinic started.

The receptionist's hair was strained back from her 'shut' face and she said she wouldn't promise anything. Ungraciously, she allowed us to wait. How perspectives change! Instead of feeling nervous about facing another biopsy I was keyed up, praying that I would be fitted in. A gleam of hope: the consultant radiologist passed through the waiting area. He stopped to talk to us, nodded sympathetically when I explained the mistake I had made, then disappeared through a swing door.

'You'll be seen,' said Erwin sagely and I was. In my relief after the uncomfortable test was over I suddenly felt very faint. The consultant radiologist summoned tea for me and urged me not to leave until I felt better. On Monday I will get a definitive result.

Looking back I see this period of uncertainty as extremely difficult and it was unfortunate that it was accidentally prolonged. At the time I didn't notice that I was finding support from writing but it was, in fact, enormously helpful – a release to describe what was happening and let out my feelings into my notebook. Working on my long narrative poem, later to be called 'Voicebox', was perhaps even more important. During this time I developed and drafted one of the most problematic sections of the poem – problematic because it was concerned with racial prejudice and because the incident had to fit into the canvas of the narrative and not swamp it. It was also hard to write because it was based on a real event but absorbing myself in it took me far away from my fear.

The other activities I've mentioned were also very helpful and I specially enjoyed treats. Even so I was under tremendous stress for weeks. This might have been lessened a little if I'd been better informed about breast cancer and the current treatments for it. I wish I'd known the prognosis for breast cancer caught at an early stage is now so good. However, I think reading up about cancer or phoning helplines at this stage might well have made me more anxious and apprehensive. The hero of Jerome K. Jerome's *Three Men In A Boat* read a medical dictionary and discovered he had the symptoms of every single illness except housemaid's knee!

CHAPTER TWO

Diagnosis

2nd February 2000

On Monday the consultant radiologist gave me the result of the second biopsy, told me without frills that I had breast cancer – grade one, the lowest order, but it's still cancer. As he spoke I saw a gun on each of his shoulders, their nozzles pointed straight at me, ready to fire. It shot through my head that I would never feel safe again, never *be* safe again. This was the end of any reasonable life. Layer on layer of fear submerged me. Today I'm wondering why I'd assumed cancer was something that happened to other people, why I'd written at the end of this year's diary a reminder to get another check up in 2002 as if there was no doubt that I would be healthy, free. My body is apparently fit but now I've been told it's not, I feel as if the cancer is worming through it, drawing me down into an underworld of illness, a world in which I'm unable to think or write, sinking into a mine of pain, into death…

Later I discovered that many people hear the news that they have cancer as a death sentence whatever they are told about the prognosis.

I was half crying, half furious at the attack on my life as we sat waiting for nearly an hour to see the surgeon. He was quiet-mannered, sympathetic but to the point. He told me he could feel the lump although it was very small and far below the surface. I wanted to disbelieve him. I wanted the cancer to be made up; I wanted to be angry with doctors and nurses. But this was decision time and shocked as I was I gathered my wits and concentrated on the course of action. At the beginning of the consultation I was under the impression that a lumpectomy, removing a part of the breast, would deal with the problem but – another shock – I was offered the choice of a mastectomy. The thought of losing a breast was terrible but my mind fastened onto a single idea: safety. It shone in my head like a huge neon sign. From the information I was given I was quickly sure that a mastectomy offered the most protection and said so. The surgeon and the breast cancer nurse both insisted I think about my decision overnight. On the way home Erwin said: 'I didn't think I should state any opinion but I'm very relieved you want to have a mastectomy because I'm certain it's the safest course of action.'

Once in the house I sobbed and sobbed. I started to make a cup of tea but almost dropped a cup as I took it off the hook in the cupboard. In a squall of fury I shouted at Erwin and threw it across the kitchen. It fell on the floor by the fridge and broke. Words screamed silently inside me: 'Why me? I will cease to be a whole person. How shocking to lose an outer visible part of my body. The breast – a symbol of feminity. I'm going to die.' Then I felt sorry I'd destroyed a cup I liked.

Among the things I'll never forget from Monday is the kindness of two close friends. First there was the message Mimi had left on the answerphone just before she went out to teach. Aware that I would need a lot of support if cancer was diagnosed she'd said: 'I was hoping to talk to you before I left. I want you to know I'm there for you and you can phone me at any time.' She has plenty of difficulties of her own to cope with but she'd even left me a phone number where I could reach her in between her two classes. I was very touched by her thoughtfulness but I didn't want to disturb her while she was in the middle of working. I left a tearful message on her home answerphone.

I had promised to phone Ruth and tell her the results when I got home. Slightly more composed after drinking a cup of tea, I dialled her number and managed to tell her the diagnosis before bursting into tears. She said: 'If you'll allow me I really would like to come and see you.' Twenty minutes later she was here and hugging me. We sat beside my books in the quiet of the poetry room, where I run my writing workshops, for maybe a couple of hours. Her presence, affection and reassurance as I cried and repeated my fears over and over, gradually calmed me.

The next day – yesterday – I was still quite clear about the decision I'd made. One or two friends urged me to get another opinion, look at other possibilities but I simply can't. This is partly because I feel convinced by the decision we've made, partly because I'm too emotionally and physically exhausted to cope with other uncertain ideas. I found it extremely comforting when Dilys, another very good friend, said she absolutely agreed with my decision. I'm relieved too that we have private health insurance and that by yesterday afternoon a plan of action was set up. I also find it reassuring to know that the operation would have been no later than next week if I'd stayed with the National Health Service.

Today I'm not in quite such a state of shock. I can see there is every reason to believe the cancer will be removed even though I keep sliding off this belief into a mire of terror and have to hoist myself back onto it or be hoisted back by Erwin. Things haven't been helped by the computer breaking down. It was affected by a short power cut on Monday evening. Erwin was unable to make it work and Ben, my son, who looks after it, is far away on holiday in Kerala. Not having access to my everyday technology has added to my sense of everything falling apart. However, I've managed to focus sufficiently to do some administrative work on Erwin's computer: sending a letter to everyone in my Reading and Writing Process workshop, postponing the workshop that should be taking place in two weeks. I've also started putting together notes which need to be sent in for a 'Writing for Self-Discovery' weekend course I'm co-tutoring in November.

In my head one voice is saying: how on earth do you imagine you'll be running that course? But another voice is saying: the course is part of my life and I'm going to hold onto the belief I'll be living it. Which is worse – the operation or the fear that it won't get rid of the cancer? Am I a coward? I made the mistake of reading a leaflet about cancer and in less than five minutes I felt as if I'd passed through every stage of the disease as it recurred and spread to other parts of my body. I was already at the gates of death, taut with terror. Yet the words came into my head: you go down and you come up. I must hold onto the idea of each moment as a 'moving on'.

I wish I wasn't putting such a strain on Erwin. I am afraid the breast cancer nurse, who is coming again tomorrow, will give me more information that will worry me. I have to hang onto the thought of friends and the relatives and friends of people I know who have survived for years and years after breast cancer. I owe it to myself to manage my panic and to make this a life experience not a death experience; to concentrate on possibilities; to grab every moment of life I can; to use what has happened for writing, to include the awfulnesses but also the plusses. I mustn't forget the moments of joy: the sun lying in swathes on the grass, the sharp clean cut of the air, the disc of the sun on water. I must keep the words that came into my head about the snowdrops I saw in a garden when we walked to the shops a couple of hours ago. I think it's the starting point of a poem.

The Snowdrops

Drops of life on this distressed afternoon. Everything grey – the concrete frontage with miserable sticks like bunches of deadness. The small white bell heads could be gathered together – could be layers pressed to my breast – could fill the space that will be left by my missing breast. These drops are not drops. The weak heads are not weak – not drooping, not dropping. They are hanging bells with thin rims of green on their delicate undersides. They have pushed through the lumpy earth and stand unmoved by the thrusting wind, the bites of cold air. They are stronger than cones of buddleia, than the can-can poppy – a brazen girl kicking. Very small, they bend but do not give way, they refuse winter, silently they remind me it can end.

Erwin and I have discussed telling his cousin about my illness. She's taken on the role of mothering me which I find difficult. She has a bit of a gloomy doomy view of life but her generosity is touching and I think she's lonely. I go along with her as far as I can. However, she considers herself an expert on illness and medical matters. I can already hear her querying every decision we've made, pounding us with alternatives. If she's given the news she'll want to get on the next train; will arrive with cakes, fruit, her swamping warmth and a hundred instructions. I simply couldn't cope. We've decided not to tell her until after the operation, though it seems cruel. It's silly but I feel as though she is someone who might take a half-full bottle and tip it until it empties out. What a marvellous relief from tension laughter is!

3rd February

Yesterday evening I ran my monthly Prose and Poetry Workshop and was really pleased I'd done so. I was able to concentrate while we read work by members of the group and during the detailed discussion we had afterwards. Running the group took me out of myself for a couple of hours. I decided in advance I would say nothing about my operation – that it would be too disturbing and distracting both for the group and me. I want to believe that I'll be able to run the next workshop at the beginning of March. I intend to do it if I possibly can.

The breast cancer nurse has been to see me for a second time and I've learnt more about my illness. She explained that it was possible the cancer had spread further, that it was most unlikely to have spread far and that there were treatments which would make me very safe. The exact situation would not be known until tests were done on samples after the operation. Of course this raised my fears higher again but she reassured me that I would survive, that my illness was treatable. I have no alternative but to be patient. I know I must focus on getting over one hurdle at a time.

This afternoon I saw Kate with whom I've had counsel-ling/therapy once a month and also a monthly massage for several years. The insights I've gained into myself and the coping mechanisms I've learnt have been invaluable in helping me become a stronger person. Kate suggested techniques to help me deal with the coming week, in particular visualizations. The main one was to close my eyes and re-experience a difficulty in breathing I once had and then to picture myself managing it, calming it until it eased and I relaxed. This fear about breathing mushroomed from the memory of a sore throat and a feeling I was about to choke when I was coming round from an operation some years ago. While trying out the visualization I remem-bered I had in fact dealt with this discomfort well, telling myself to breathe shallowly and that the sensation would wear off, which it did.

I've found it somehow reassuring to discover that the fears that have dominated me this week are very similar to the fears other people go through in this situation. In a card on Monday and on the phone today John was very sympathetic and caring. John is a close friend, a poet and writer, who has spent the last few years doing some ground-breaking work in writing residencies with dementia sufferers, helping them express their feelings and thoughts. He lives in Yorkshire but he's attached to Stirling University and spends much of his working time in Scotland. He ran the Littlewood Press in the 1980s and was my first poetry publisher. I am aware how very much I need the support and affection of the main people in my life. I'm lucky I'm getting it. Erwin, of course, is helping me all the time.

4th February

I was irritable and slow this morning because I've had to take a sleeping pill or half a sleeping pill each night this week. However, it cheered me to get a request today from someone who heard me give a poetry reading a few years ago. She wants me to read at a poetry festival in May which makes me feel that life, and in particular my poetry life, will continue. The thought of losing all this because I'm set apart by illness has been very depressing. I've spoken to Mimi two or three times this week. Like Ruth she's been amazingly supportive and today I received a card from her. Inside she's written: 'Just to say I love you very much and to wish you the very best for the operation and your hospital stay and for the best of all recoveries.' Her message made me cry.

My throat's a bit sore and my nose has been runny on and off so I've felt worried that I might be getting a cold. I phoned the hospital about this and a nurse reassured me that a minor cold wouldn't stand in the way of the operation. Before lunch we walked along Waterfall Walk, a strip of parkland at the end of our road which runs by the small river. The area, which is wooded by the water, has been left more or less wild. Being with untamed nature always makes me feel better. This evening we made the weekly soup. Most of it goes in portions to our ninety-year-old sweet-natured neighbour, Adrian Taylor. It was extraordinarily therapeutic making the soup this time, relishing the smell of it cooking, knowing it was life-sustaining. Enough has gone into the freezer to keep Adrian going for at least ten days.

In spite of these positive activities fear of the operation domi-nated me all day. Late in the evening in a state of high nervousness – I've always found hospitals frightening places – I suddenly decided to write down everything that was on my mind in my notebook. I was aware that this was something John and I had recommended to others in the journal section of the handbook, *Writing for Self-Discovery*, which we wrote together a few years ago. In fact instinctively I set myself to do one of the exercises which asks the reader to make a list of all the different feelings she/he is aware of. This is what I wrote:

What's On My Mind

I am afraid of the operation.
I am afraid they won't do the operation because I have a bit of a cold.
It will be a relief if they do the operation – even to have the fear of the operation.

I am afraid of going through another waiting period and the disease spreading.

I am afraid of the anaesthetic.

I am afraid of the period after coming round.

I am afraid that I'll have difficulty with breathing.

I am afraid of being very weak and muzzy.

I am afraid of not being in control.

I am afraid of being seen as a feeble coward.

I am afraid of the wound and the discomfort.

I am very sad I am losing one of my small breasts.

I am even afraid that they will remove the wrong breast.

I am less afraid because there is still a purple bruise on my left breast.

I am also less afraid because the surgeon will see me before the operation and I will check he knows it is the left breast.

I am afraid that although the prognosis is good they will discover that the cancer has spread more than they think.

The operation is a gateway through which I must pass and my life will be longer if I do pass through it.

I want to pass through it and I want it to be tomorrow.

I want to fight my fear.

I want to make the best use I can of the rest of my life whatever it is.

I want to write about cancer in different ways including writing poems about it – both for myself and other people.

I want and believe I will be able to do this to support myself and communicate my experience to others.

Writing this entry helped me beyond anything I could have imagined. I had tried this kind of writing before and believed in it but it was a long time since I had been in such an extreme situation. The list itself shows how writing it helped me. After I had crystallized all the terrors spinning in my mind and put them outside myself by 'dumping' them in my notebook I felt a lightening. I can remember the feeling of change as I stated definitely that the operation was a gateway I wanted to pass through. By then I was sufficiently released from fear for positive thoughts to surface. Indeed by the time I reached the end of the entry I felt a sense of uplift.

I find it difficult to sleep if something is on my mind but I did get quite a few hours' sleep that night and I'm certain it was because I'd written that notebook entry. I was awake for a while in the middle of the night but I deflected my anxiety about the following morning by thinking up some more lines about 'not telling' people about my illness. I scribbled the new lines in my diary at 2.30a.m.:

I'm not going to tell her because…

she's sanctimonious as a Victorian steeple

she's a miserable old martyr

she has less compassion than a hawthorn, and is never crowned with white blossom.

CHAPTER THREE

Hospital

5th February 2000, 9.15p.m.

I have gone through the gates today. It's been the easiest recovery I've had from any operation. The anaesthetist – a young and lively woman – had a delightful manner. I'm less weak than I expected – just have to cope with the recovery and my fear that they discover the cancer is worse than they thought. There's nothing I can do except concentrate on positives but I feel I've managed the day quite well. Of course I've been so supported by Erwin, the medical people and my friends.

> I was amazed and triumphant that I felt strong enough to write a few words in my notebook on the same day as the operation, that my fears about it were now phantoms. We'd got up early in order to be at the hospital by 7a.m. As we drove away from the house I had something of the sense of making an early start on a holiday, an adventure – and looking back the rest of the year could be certainly described as an adventure with many endurance tests.
>
> The anaesthetist had insisted I would be able to eat lunch around two o'clock. I didn't believe her but not wanting to disappoint her enthusiasm I chose from the menu. The preliminaries before the operation were very few as the paperwork had been

done on Wednesday and I was given no injection in advance. All this added to the general informality and lessened my dread.

I came round easily from the anaesthetic and though I didn't eat any lunch I had tea and toast around 3p.m. Erwin came to see me and later I enjoyed supper. I was so relieved I even phoned Ruth and John and talked to each of them for a minute or two. It was trying having two drains attached to me and, of course, I was very weak but I managed to get out of bed to go to the loo.

6th February

The nurse in charge last night was Aziz from the Gulf. He told me he liked working for a few years in one country and then moving on. He wanted to know if my name, Schneider, was German. I explained that Erwin was a refugee from Vienna and that he'd come to England with his mother to escape from Hitler six months before World War Two. This conversation made me feel I was back in a normal world where one met new people and learnt about their lives and careers. Aziz was also kind and practical. I woke up feeling shaky around one in the morning and my wounded breast area was painful. By the time I'd made my way to the loo I felt nauseous as well. He gave me an injection and I went back to sleep.

When Erwin came yesterday he'd been without any heating at home because the gas boiler's pilot light had gone out. Yet another thing to contend with. However, in the evening the gas company told him over the phone how to relight it and he was proud of himself for managing to do this. I was pleased and relieved to hear of his success when he called me.

This morning Ruth came to visit me and brought daffodil buds. I looked at them standing in a tall vase and it seemed to me that their heads were turned towards us as if calling. The daffodils are mixed with stems of delicate leaves which look dark green against the cream of the wall. They're thin as willow leaves but not as long – eucalyptus maybe – and they make me think of a Chinese painting. Ruth had hardly gone when the good-natured breast cancer nurse appeared. She got me out of bed to start doing exercises for my arm and breast. In less than a minute I felt faint and had to lie down but I'll be conscientious about doing these exercises.

At lunch-time Ben phoned from Kerala. Instinctively I hadn't told him about the investigation because he's highly strung. When he went away – a few days before the diagnosis – Erwin and I discussed telling him but decided it was pointless to worry him when he was going so far especially as it was very possible there might be nothing seriously wrong. However, he'd arranged to phone us this weekend and we realized that now he would feel information had been withheld if we kept the news until he came home. Besides we had reassuring information about the prognosis and the operation was over. We also knew that Pogle, his partner, who was with him, would be supportive.

It was such a surprise to hear Ben's voice in my room as clear as if he was standing beside me. It simply hadn't occurred to me that he would try to reach me in hospital and it was a huge lift that he wanted to talk to me. Erwin had explained the situation to him but he was rather shocked and upset at the beginning of our conversation. However, he calmed down when he could hear how well I'd come through the operation and I assured him, as Erwin had, that the outlook was good. I told him I intended to make the most of the rest of my life whatever it was and that he wasn't to waste any of his holiday worrying. It sounded as if the pair of them had been having a fantastic time: the totally different culture and landscape – the noise of people, the strange smells, the sea, the inland waters and wildlife.

Erwin spent all the afternoon with me. When he left he reappeared almost immediately with Vicki Golding. She'd been visiting someone in the hospital and he'd bumped into her on the way out. I've known Vicki for over thirty years but not very closely. Our paths hadn't crossed for a long time but she'd been in my thoughts as news had reached me about ten days ago that her partner had collapsed and died on a plane on the way home from Australia. I'd intended to get hold of her address and write to her but hadn't because of my own problems. She was also on my mind because she'd had breast cancer. I was very touched that she wanted to come to see me at a time when she was in a state of shock and bereavement. I quickly told her I'd heard about

Barry's death and saw the look of relief on her face that she hadn't got to tell me the news. We talked about cancer – both mine and her past experience – and she told me about her feelings on the plane journey back to England, her grief. The conversation was very open, and I found it supportive and moving. She's promised to pop in and see me again.

7th February

In the middle of last night I was aware of the flatness of my left breast. I felt bereft especially as I've had no womb since my hysterectomy in 1982. I found myself picturing Modigliani women and I saw myself nullified. I didn't think I'd be able to sleep but I dropped off immediately.

Poetry Please yesterday afternoon on Radio 4 had two poems I'd requested at least three years ago: my friend Grevel Lindop's gorgeous 'Summer Pudding' and Anne Stevenson's haunting 'In A Tunnel of Summers'. Erwin taped the programme for me and although I was tired and spaced out I managed to focus on it fairly well this morning. The subject was the senses. It felt good to be mentioned as poet Myra Schneider.

8th February

Yesterday was a very long day and I was extremely tired by the end of it – I'd been more or less awake from 3a.m. I'm stronger, of course, but also more conscious of the change in my body and very up and down. I lay tearful in the early morning, extremely aware of the absence of my breast especially as some of the dressing has been removed. I didn't feel a sense of loss when I had a hysterectomy – only relief that I wouldn't have any more heavy periods. A breast is such a visible sign of femininity, so often painted and written about. I keep remembering being told: 'I love your small breasts.' I thought of breasts feeding babies and I remembered how as an adolescent I'd wished I wasn't female, didn't have breasts, periods. Partly this was a fear of sexuality.

It was a long time before I consciously enjoyed the feeling that I was a woman.

Dilys came to see me and although my concentration was still limited it was great to see her and also to talk about two anthologies of poetry by women that she and I are involved in editing. As a present Dilys brought me *Repair*, C.K. Williams' new collection. Slowly I've read and re-read 'Train' and 'Ice'. The detail is very graphic and I love the distances the poems travel and the emotion they carry. I'm a bit more focused this morning and can feel this is powerful writing. What a wonderfully titled book to receive as a get well present.

8/9th February (middle of night)

The world of hospital has its own rhythms which I'm becoming more attuned to. Each day I think I'm managing the system better. Mimi came to see me and again it was lovely to have lots of talk that had nothing to do with illness.

The Bath

The comfort of the bath this morning was extraordinary even though it had to be shallow so that the wound didn't get wet. The water was warm, softening my back and buttocks, all the tension in my muscles melting like a miracle, the sense of cleansing, the lavender of the bath essence filling my nostrils, an overwhelming sense of release, a blessing – surely a poem here? I remembered the first bath I had a few days after Ben was born: the salt in the water, a feeling of letting go, of being a baby myself. The joy, the relief of this morning's bath was so intense you simply couldn't experience it if you hadn't been through an ordeal. Money couldn't buy such a gift. In some way this terrible experience has enhanced my life.

I have to find a way of assimilating, feeling safe with my new shape. The breast cancer nurse came in again today to see how I was getting on. She wanted me to look at the wound, said I must come to terms with it. I immediately felt ill and slightly faint. She didn't insist when I said I wasn't up to it but suggested it would be better if I looked at it before I left the hospital, that anyway it would need a new dressing by the end of the week.

9th February

I remember I woke up earlyish and in the dark I gingerly touched my chest, recognized my new shape and cried. It was a relief to allow the tears, to be alone with my feelings in the stillness. Words, images started to form in my head for a poem. It was calming to be gathering and sorting them. About six – just before the nurses started the first round of the morning – I began drafting the poem in my notebook. Trying to work brought it home to me how foggy-headed I still was but I was determined to get the words down.

There were constant interruptions: temperature to be taken, tea, breakfast, having another shallow bath, the room being cleaned, the phone going. It was nearly eleven by the time I'd managed to reach the end of the poem. By this time I was sitting on a chair. Tired but with a feeling of considerable satisfaction, even though I was already doubtful about the ending, I put my notebook down on the bed. A few moments later the surgeon came into the room. 'How are you?' he asked.

'I've just finished drafting a poem,' I replied. This is what I'd written:

Today There Is Time
to think about the way life
opens, clams, parts,

to savour remembered rosemaries,
spreading purples, white

pricked edges of hope.
Today there is time to breathe in

the silken stillness of being
with myself, take in the loss

of my left breast, to lay
my nervous palm softly

as a bird's wing across
my new plain, allow

tears to fall yet rejoice
that the surgeon scraped cells

of death. Today there's time
to merge with the writer of *Repair*

as he 'longs painfully out' from
the train, to be the hare

he sees in the rime in the scrub.
Today there is time to travel

the meanings of repair, put them?*
in words that open parachutes.

*Note: Question mark because I didn't like 'put them'.

The repeated line: 'Today there is time' was like a banister to lean on. Although I knew the draft wasn't quite right I felt sure it was a real poem. I also knew writing it had helped me to cope both physically and emotionally with my single-breasted chest. When the breast nurse came again at the end of the week I was able to look at the wound calmly. I made one or two changes to the poem over the next few days but couldn't think how to change 'put them'.

11th February

Yesterday evening I found myself thinking of Veronica. In the last week my admiration for the courage and strength she showed during the illness which killed her has grown much greater. I think I'm being positive about my illness but isn't that because at some level I believe I'm going to live? I first met Veronica when she joined one of my poetry workshops. A cheerful middle-aged woman, she often made lively and intelligent comments in the group. However, she was also lacking in confidence about her own work and usually brought unfinished poems with many crossings out on scraps of paper. After a time she left me to attend workshops in central London but I bumped into her from time to time. Then I heard she'd been diagnosed with liver cancer and that it was terminal. Chemotherapy prolonged her life for a year and a half and she astonished everyone by becoming much more focused and positive during this time. She finished off several poems, was realistic about her prognosis, but continued to take part in everything she could. I spoke to her on the phone sometimes and occasionally saw her at events.

Lying in bed I pictured myself walking arm in arm with her at the launch of my collection of poetry, *The Panic Bird*, and how enthusiastic she was about the evening. It's true she had a supportive net of people round her which included Dilys, who was constant and selfless in her kindness, but her fortitude and determination came from within herself. I thought of the moving reading she gave at the Torriano Meeting House in November, my realization that I wouldn't see her again. I remembered I talked to her once and sent cards. I also remembered the launch of a booklet of her poems published by Hearing Eye Press five days before her death on Christmas Day and how she listened to the taped recording which included each of us reading a poem from it.

John had to come to London to do some work and it was great to see him yesterday and talk about books and writing. However, I've been very up and down during the last twenty-four hours because I'm expecting to get the results of tests done on the cancerous material which was in my breast. It's been impossible to push the fear of death out of my head.

When the surgeon came this afternoon he told me the tumour had spread a little, passed through two nodes. He said the chances of the cancer returning were small now that I'd had the operation but to reduce them to an absolute minimum I must have follow up treatment. This would be set up by an oncologist who would prescribe the exact form of the treatment once he had the full results. These are expected at the end of next week. He spoke as though both chemotherapy and radiotherapy were a likelihood – the radiotherapy because the small cancerous area had been deep, close to my chest. It was fortunate that Mimi had already told me that chemotherapy is used as a curative. In my ignorance I'd always thought it was no more than a palliative.

It is an overwhelming relief to have information which convinces me I am not going to die in the next year, that my future will be as safe as anyone's can be. I've been in such a high state of tension I couldn't immediately – and still can't – unwind. I know I must try and be calmer, give myself time to get over the traumas of the last two weeks. I've also decided – and it feels momentous but very right – that I want to write a sequence of poems about cancer and keep this notebook going.

12th February, 4 a.m.

It is the middle of the night and I've found myself thinking again: What are the chances of cancer returning? I'm reminding myself that they're extremely small. When I was given the diagnosis I thought I'd never feel safe again – but why did I feel safe in the first place? In fact it was a false sense of safety. Now I'm grateful that I will have a high level of safety. My perspective has completely changed. I'm afraid of the follow up treatment but I shall not allow it to disturb what I intend to do any more than I can help. This is a new stage in my life.

CHAPTER FOUR

Recovery from the Operation 1

13th February 2000

I had a strong sense of let down when I came home after an operation a few years ago so I didn't expect too much yesterday. It was a cold, bright day but there were orange crocuses in the front garden and daffodil buds were just beginning to open. I hadn't noticed how much it had rained during the week and was surprised to see pools in the park behind our house. In the sun the water glinted like pieces of glass.

Because of warnings about the after-effects of removing lymph nodes I'd built up a fear that my left arm would be more or less out of action but it's not – I just mustn't lift anything heavy. I soon had the coffee grinder out and revelled in the strong aroma of coffee beans as I ground them. I savoured each mouthful of real coffee, then lay in bed for a while, not minding feeling weak – just glad to be back in my room. I wanted to smell fresh air, which I'd been cut off from for a week, so before lunch Erwin walked down the road with me. By the time we'd passed three houses I was exhausted and had to turn back but it was wonderful to feel the cold wind roughing my face, to be out of the muffled world of hospital.

In the middle of the night I woke up and began to worry about everything. Was it a good idea to continue teaching at Flightways? Would I be able to manage my writing groups, do poetry readings? The thought of making decisions and changes was overwhelming. It was also daunting to think how many friends didn't yet know about my illness. I would be a leper bearing bad news about breast cancer. Already I could hear their shocked voices, feel their shock rebound on me. The difficulties piled up in monstrous layers. The weight of them was unbearable. Eventually I put on Kate's relaxation tape – the side with visualizations. My favourite is 'The Egg of Protection' which begins by asking the listener to visualize a shade of pink flowing through her/his body and then surrounding it in an egg shape. As I listened I began to cry and I didn't try to stop myself. Kate's soothing voice as well as the visualization seemed to open me to all the distress of the last few weeks. It was almost as if she was in the room encouraging me to recognize my feelings. When the tape ended I began to feel calmer and I fell asleep.

I spoke to John on the phone this morning and told him that I'd been crying in the night. He was very sympathetic. I felt better and wanted to know what he thought about 'Today There Is Time' which I'd e-mailed him. 'This is going to be a good poem,' he said, 'but it needs more work. You've got so hooked on the idea of repair from C.K. Williams' *Repair* that the end has been invaded by his train poem.' He also pointed out that my poem began in the wrong place – needed the action first, not the reflection. He suggested it would fall naturally into two stanzas. I knew at once that he was right. He always gets to the heart of what is working, and what isn't.

When I went back to the poem the next day I wondered why I'd not thought about the direction of the poem. I now realize that at the time of drafting I could only make my way into it by echoing the train of thought which had made it possible for me to touch my chest. Once I recognized what was needed to make the poem coherent I re-structured it in less than an hour. It was during this process that the word 'tug' hit me and I finalized the last two lines. Afterwards I made only one or two very small revisions. Usually I write much more slowly than this – build up poems gradually from a series of notes, images and ideas – but the situation had demanded a different approach. Here is the poem in its final version:

Today There Is Time
to touch the silken stillness
of myself, map its landscape,
the missing left breast, to lay
my nervous palm softly
as a bird's wing across
the new plain, allow
tears to fall yet rejoice
that the surgeon scraped
away the cancer cells.

Today there is time
to contemplate the way life
opens, clams, parts, savour
its remembered rosemaries,
spreading purples, tight
white edges of hope, to travel
the meanings of repair, tug
words that open parachutes.

Later this morning, Stephen, my publisher at Enitharmon, came for coffee. He brought me flowers and it was so morale-boosting to sit talking books, poetry. He also brought the typescript of *Insisting on Yellow*, my new and selected poems, with a list of queries which he said was very small. The tangible progress of the book was very encouraging. Stephen suggested we went through his points together but I knew I wasn't clear-headed enough to focus. I promised to look at them and respond in the next few days.

14th February

Dumping: Against Cancer

Cancer the red scare word
the Gorgon fixing you with its eye word,
the big bad wolf in the wood word,
the stick it up your arse, slap it on its head,
slam shut its gobbling mouth word
the wear it as a brooch
by your missing breast word.
It's the word that coils secretly
through the house of your body,
climbs the stairs,
takes possession of each landing.
The word to crumple, spit on,
stick in the bin,
clash cymbals at until it drops its arrogance.
The word to crush with:
'you won't shrivel me
with your huff and puff,
scientific terms,
smack-happy treatments'.
The word to throw out with hallelujahs of the heart.

I feel invigorated by writing these lines, as if I've hit back at cancer and doctors. (I know doctors want to help me but deep down it doesn't feel like it. I suppose it's a bit like blaming messengers who bring bad news.) The piece is hardly subtle but maybe this is a time to slap down some unsubtle words! Would it make a short poem round the word 'cancer' – and with rhyme? I'm not sure – it might have fulfilled its purpose.

15th February

I've been thinking about safety – my fantasy that I was safe from breast cancer because my breasts were small. Total safety doesn't exist – the truth is we are all always in danger. One has to accept that – build one's own peace of mind, live creatively, make every moment as fruitful as possible – otherwise we are just wasting life. I've never felt this so strongly – the illness has given me a new, maybe a clearer perspective. It's ironic to remember that my father got it into his head when he was around eighty that he had cancer. Although he was a brilliant scientist he was completely illogical, hooking his fears around some minor blood tests, and it was a few years before he stopped talking ominously about 'his illness'. I've heard of other instances of people who became obsessed with the belief that they had cancer.

16th February

The breast cancer nurse has visited me again. On the basis of the test results she said she thought the oncologist would want me to have a mild form of chemotherapy. She also thought radiotherapy was a strong likelihood – twenty-five short treatments, one every weekday. Her description of chemotherapy – and she went into quite a lot of detail – upset and angered me. I suppose because I'm still weak it's frightening to hear about this treatment which takes months and is also debilitating. There is something repulsive about the idea of attacking the entire body in order to kill any possible stray destructive cells. I am worried that the treatment will interfere with giving readings and running writing courses. Of course for my own protection I have no choice so somehow I must prepare myself. All the fear and tension I've felt round this has rubbed off on Erwin. This afternoon he lost his temper with an assistant in the chemist shop.

17th February

I have received a wonderful letter from Elizabeth Bewick. It's ironic to think I did a reading with her and stayed with her a few weeks ago without knowing that this straight-backed woman, who's over eighty and full of character, has survived both breast cancer and bowel cancer. Her letter was so sympathetic, so understanding of exactly the kind of fears I have been going through. She explained that she was only telling me her own history to show me that I would survive. When I was with her I was struck by the fact that she had an extraordinary capacity to enjoy life – the small things. She'd put a bathrobe in my bedroom so that we could have the fun of eating breakfast before we dressed and breakfast itself consisted of goodies which began with a basket of strawberries.

What's On My Mind

I am terrified of facing chemotherapy.

I am dreading feeling sick and being out of action or partly out of action.

I am afraid of my hair thinning and falling out.

I feel ill just thinking about this treatment.

I feel upset that I have to think about this while I'm recovering from the operation.

I feel overwhelmed that I have so much to contend with.

I feel worried because a tooth has broken and the crown has come off the tooth next to it.

I feel strung up about changing or cancelling work fixtures.

I feel bothered about putting other people out.

I feel ashamed that I swore and threw my clipboard on the floor and made Erwin very tense when the battery ran out while we were listening to his tape recording of the surgeon explaining my results.

I feel it's the last straw to know I might have to undergo radiotherapy too.

I don't want to give up.

I want to retire from Flightways – it would be a relief.

I find it daunting even to think about dealing with this.
I want to focus on doing things day by day.
I want to accept it will take a long time to sort everything out.
I want to put my safety first.
I feel better if I think about what I've already managed to get through and do.

> Again, dumping my jumble of fears and other feelings into my notebook was a tremendous release. Once on paper they stopped going round and round in my head and I began to be more positive and focused.

18th February

I've been asked to write a piece for the 'Poets I Go Back To' series in *The North* magazine. This is gratifying and, although I still don't feel very together, it's straightforward in that it doesn't need the careful reading and analysis required for writing a review so I'm going to do it. I shall enjoy the freedom of being able to include exactly what I want to. The only difficulty is choosing which of my favourites to focus on. Before I dressed this morning I re-read 'Lines Written a Few Miles Above Tintern Abbey'. This poem of Wordsworth's is ingrained in me and especially:

> And I have felt
> A presence that disturbs me with the joy
> Of elevated thoughts; a sense sublime
> Of something far more deeply interfused,
> Whose dwelling is the light of setting suns,
> And the round ocean, and the living air,
> And the blue sky, and in the mind of man,
> A motion and a spirit, that impels
> All thinking things, all objects of all thought,
> And rolls through all things.

Both the philosophy and the descriptions of nature had a profound influence on me when I was about seventeen.

Friends have been so good about keeping in touch and seeing people makes life feel more normal. It was lovely to have Angie here for a simple supper yesterday. She did speech therapy sessions at Flightways for several years and as we shared several clients we often pooled our expertise and experience. Last night I told her that I was thinking of leaving Flightways. We discussed the fact that I probably wouldn't be fit to return there maybe till late in the year. Then after a few months I'd be due to retire and that as far as my most needy students were concerned, I'd *disappear* twice which would do more harm than good. Angie has a very calm, sympathetic manner and going over all this helped me crystallize my decision that I must give up my work there now.

It will be a wrench to leave people like Abdul whose main disability is deafness. He started attending Flightways years ago when he was in his twenties. I found he had no speech, couldn't use any signing system, couldn't read, write or recognize letters. It was clear he had some memory problems but also areas of considerable intelligence, that he was very motivated, had a sense of fun and a strong personality. With back-up from others I've managed to teach him a certain amount of simple signing and a basic vocabulary of about two hundred words. He enjoys writing, can read simple stories and answer questions about them. I am afraid my departure means he will get much less input.

Not long after Angie went I found Erwin searching tensely round the house for his credit card. I persuaded him to phone Sainsbury's where he'd used it this morning but it hadn't been found. I urged him to get it cancelled.

'Then I'll have no card for several days,' he muttered, 'and anyway I'm sure it's in the house somewhere.' By now I felt weak and exhausted but I reminded myself that he was low, on antibiotics for toothache, and that the strain of the last few weeks had taken its toll. Around ten o'clock, as if defeated in battle, he gave in.

19th February

This afternoon I finally managed to make a small start on the article 'Poets I Go Back To'. I was in a bit of a state at first because I had to do it on Erwin's computer with different software but I calmed down once I'd produced a couple of paragraphs. What I'm writing is not startlingly original or clever but it is a recognition of some of my deepest poetic influences and I'm going to take the opportunity to make a comment on contemporary poetry. It will be such a relief when Ben is back from Kerala and gets my computer going again.

All during this week I've added lines to 'I'm Not Going To Tell Her' and now I've turned it into a poem. It's been fun to do, a way of keeping things in proportion. Erwin is going to phone his cousin up and tell her 'the news' so that I shall not have to endure the weight of her sympathy. I've also decided to stagger telling friends who don't yet know about my illness as this will be less stressful and I've realized it will be easier to tell them in letters.

20th February

There's a swelling round my lymph gland and the wound feels very tight. I first became aware of this when we went out for a walk yesterday and, although I remembered the breast cancer nurse saying such swellings were a possibility, I began to feel anxious, even slightly faint. During the night the soreness of my chest and arm was worse, painful enough to stop me sleeping. In the end I took a paracetamol, put on Kate's relaxation tape and managed to drop off. This morning the swelling under my arm was more visible so I phoned the hospital. I spoke to a nurse who was reassuring and asked the surgeon to ring me. He said it was nothing to worry about and that he would be looking at the swelling when he saw me in his clinic on Tuesday.

Ben and Pogle are back from Kerala. They were very jet-lagged and I told Ben not to rush over here but give himself time to come to. Nevertheless he was here within a couple of days and had my computer working in next to no time. I was touched that he wanted to see for himself how I was. He brought me a wooden box with different compartments and a carved swivel lid as well as spices, some of which I've put in the box. I'm so pleased to have my own machine in action again in my workroom. It feels like a step towards normality.

21st February

I'm writing this while waiting to see the oncologist at the Nuffield Hospital in Enfield. John thought the poem 'I'm Not Going To Tell Her' only worked as therapy. I was disappointed because I'd had fun with the images, also worked hard with them and I really thought it was more than that. In fact I felt reluctant to relinquish the poem so I sent it to Mimi for another opinion. On the phone yesterday she said she thinks it is a poem but that I need to make it more extravagant and humorous, to take the images further. That sounded right to me and in the middle of last night some new images jumped into my head. I think I've more or less got the poem now.

> Later on when *The North* accepted the poem I made a change in the first verse to bring the images more in line with one another and I did one or two tightenings but substantially the poem was finished. Here is the final version:

I'm Not Going To Tell Her

because she's splintery as a weather-beaten fence,
sanctimonious as a Victorian steeple,
because she's a lifetime member of the Guild of Job's
Comforters,
because she'll take a half-full bottle and tip it till it trickles
out.

I'm not going to tell her
because she has less compassion than a hawthorn bush
and is never crowned with wild white blossom,
because generosity – its red berry juice – never sweetens her
sentences.

I'm not going to tell her
because she's boring as water biscuits, as a dripping tap,
because she rattles medical information like a large bottle of
tablets
and permanently wears a tense prefect's badge,

because her doomladen voice,
inevitable as a steam roller, flattens me into insignificance,
buries me deep in its slough of despond, because
she's not in touch with her own feelings so how can she
connect with mine?

I've finished C.K. Williams' *Repair*. The writing is highly keyed emotionally, the language vigorous and wide ranging, the thought complex. The poems often travel a long way through extraordinary shifts. It feels like my book for the year – even the title.

23rd February

Nothing's arranged for today so the day is my oyster – I can open it any way I like. Even though my body is changed and my whole system out of synch – sometimes I feel very empty, sometimes very full – I'm aware of a sense of uplift, that life has a special value, that I want to catch every precious drop of it. Spring returning, all the flowers in the house from friends, feed into my elation.

On Monday the oncologist still didn't have all my results so the only thing definitely decided is that I must take Tamoxifen for five years and have twenty-five sessions of radiotherapy. The treatment will take place at a clinic on Harley Street and will begin immediately after we've taken the holiday in Nice which we booked last autumn. I'm so pleased the oncologist agreed, indeed encouraged us to go on this holiday. There's still a possibility I won't have to undergo chemotherapy at all but I'm not counting on it. At least I have time to continue building up my strength. When I saw the surgeon he said my wound was healing well and he confirmed that the swelling and the tightness and soreness are to be expected.

Yesterday it felt good to be writing notes about the Second Light poetry competition which I judged in November. One of my aims during these past weeks has been to recover sufficiently to go and talk at the adjudication this coming Saturday afternoon. I feel I can make it. Dilys, who has an amazing amount of energy, started the Second Light Network in 1995. Its purpose is to bring older women poets together and promote women's poetry in general. Dilys contacted me as a writing tutor when she was setting up the network and it was through this that we met and became friends. I was interested in the idea because, although there has been a great outburst of women's poetry in the last twenty years, men still hold the most powerful positions in the poetry world. I also liked the idea because most attention goes – as it does in all fields – to the gimmicky, the sensational, the new and the trendy.

Erwin has spoken to his cousin and her reaction was exactly as the poem had predicted. She interrogated him about who performed the operation, sounding all the time suspicious – as if she knew a great many surgeons and had special knowledge of their capabilities. She seemed totally oblivious of the fact that the operation had been performed two and a half weeks ago, that it was pointless now to discuss whether it had been performed by a suitable surgeon. When she heard I might have to have chemotherapy she pronounced in a voice of doom that my hair would fall out and that I'd be sick. Then she barked: 'Myra must go to the best cancer hospital.' Erwin said firmly: 'This is a routine procedure so we don't need Harrods.' Then he held the receiver at some distance from his ear while at the top of her voice she argued herself to a standstill in a mixture of German and English. There was another volley when he said I wasn't strong enough to see her but Erwin held firm. I am sure she genuinely *wants* to be kind, is convinced that she is being helpful but she hits the wrong note every time. Even when she gives us a present she delivers a series of abrupt instructions as if we are too stupid to make best use of it. A stroke of luck: she's going to Vienna in ten days and will be there for at least two months to stay with an aged cousin who has broken a leg. I believe this cousin is quite a tyrant so there might be something of a battle!

I found it funny that she had behaved exactly in line with the poem and yet I panicked – maybe she really did have special information – and I felt more frightened than ever about the possibility of chemotherapy. I phoned the Breast Cancer Care Helpline and a sympathetic counsellor told me there were pills that controlled sickness following chemotherapy, that it was unlikely all my hair would fall out, that the little she knew about the clinic I was with was positive and to phone again if another demon crossed my path.

Vicki came to see me and brought three hyacinths in tight bud in a bowl. They made me think of small pointed breasts. Vicki has written a book with my friend, Sheila, and her daughter, Jo, who had ovarian cancer. She was feeling pleased because the book, *44½ Choices you can make if you have cancer* has now found a publisher. She also told me she's kept a diary for years and that she's found writing in it particularly supportive during difficult times.

CHAPTER FIVE

Recovery from the Operation 2

26th February 2000

I dressed earlier this morning so I must be feeling stronger but I'm again very conscious of my changed shape – the absence of my breast and the shock of having cancer has hit me all over again. Adjusting is an ongoing process. But now I feel delighted, triumphant even, because I made it to the adjudication of the competition. It was only possible because Erwin took me and because the venue is less than half an hour's drive away. I was greeted with warmth and, although I felt dazed, I spoke about the competition for a few minutes, then stayed on to hear the first part of the reading. It's uplifting to take part in an event again. When we arrived home I had tea and toast. I took the tea up to bed and looked at the poem I'm writing round the snowdrops I saw before the operation. I was only going to read through the draft but the moment I looked at it, I saw how to move on from the point where I was stuck this morning so I carried on working for half an hour. Then I closed my eyes and listened to harp music. I'm getting

27th February, Afternoon

Mixed-up Feelings

I feel lopsided.
I feel a freak with parts of my body missing.
I feel every other woman has a perfect two-breasted agile body.
I feel like an ancient creaking vehicle.
I feel I have entered a new phase of my life.
I feel I have permission to concentrate on what I most want to do.
I feel I can't stand any more strain.
I feel lucky to be alive.
I feel maimed.
I feel glad science has gone far enough to diagnose my illness early.
I feel glad it has the means to make me safer.
I feel lopping off a breast is primitive.
I feel more appreciation of the good things in life.
I feel recuperation is a drag.
I feel afraid that cancer will somehow find its way back in.
I feel elated by what I'm managing to do.
I feel overwhelmed by the different shocks and difficulties.
I feel doors have shut.
I feel other doors have opened.
I feel I've been slapped down.
I feel I've moved forward in life.

Flow-Writing

I feel doors have shut and I am locked in an airless room. A great weight of books and blankets is pressing down on me. I want to get up but how can I throw off everything that's holding me down? Doesn't anyone understand how weak I feel, how tangled up in a web with that spider treatment waiting to snare me? I don't want to be here. I want to walk miles and miles over the South Downs and hear larks and see waves of wind passing through green wheat. Can I wriggle out? Can I shrink everything I hate by barking, by screaming with laughter, by jumping up and down? Scarecrow, I'm a scarecrow – but I could unlatch, throw everything open, come upon butterflies.

> Although my feelings remained 'mixed up' right through these pieces I can remember both the sense of release and the feeling of energy gathering, spurring me on as I wrote them.

28th February

Yesterday I managed the twenty-five minute walk round the park for the first time. It was sufficiently spring-like to stop and sit on a bench. I so enjoyed being out. In the evening Ben and Pogle came. Ben arrived with food and produced a delicious meal. He took an enormous number of photographs in Kerala and brought two or three packets of them to show us. There were pictures of palm treescapes, the sea and inland waterways, very green hills, the hotel they stayed at in a nature reserve, also of the old town of Cochin which is where he bought the spices he's shared with me.

I feel more normal today. My head feels clearer, my legs stronger, my chest and armpit less wounded. I've done virtually a morning's work – written the notes for my writing group on Wednesday evening and finished the draft of 'Snowdrops'. I started with the few lines I wrote in my notebook but I've done much more planning and drafting than I did for 'Today There Is Time'.

Snowdrops

As I stare at the small
white heads, their circular bed
set in a bald frontage,
the afternoon swells
with distress. I imagine picking,
imagine pressing layers
of green-rimmed petals
to my chest to cover
the emptiness which will shout
when I lose my left breast.

Though they look weak
beneath a bush's crude
black spread of branches
these are not drops, crystals,
bells that ring thinly,
not hangdog ninnies,
timid girls running out of breath.

They have heaved through
weighty clay lumps,
speared freezing air
to bloom without summer's prop –
are more daring
than can-can poppies,
fiercer than the swimming
open-mouthed fear that wants
to devour me. They stand
uncowed by the north wind,
its sudden bluster, cruel bite.
And as I move on each flower
fills me like an annunciation.

2nd March

Resources that have helped me

1. Writing: my notebook and poems.

2. Listening to the radio.

3. Visualizations, especially Kate's relaxation tape.

4. Friends coming to see me and talking to friends on the phone.

5. Enjoying small things: signs of spring, flowers and cards I've received.

6. Hearing about positive experiences of cancer.

7. Counselling with Kate.

8. Visiting nearby friends and feeling strong enough to begin going out.

9. Noticing the progress I'm making.

Yesterday afternoon I had a session with Kate. We talked about my recovery; I told her that although I could face the wound and that writing 'Today There Is Time' has been a great help, I still avoid looking at it even though it's not so raw now. I said I disliked dressing and undressing, that the moment of taking clothes off feels very uncomfortable. On the other hand I find baths marvellously comforting. I also told Kate that I'm terribly aware of being lopsided and different from other women and that although some of the numbness has worn off, the whole area of my chest and upper arm is sore and sometimes I have needle-like shooting pains in my arm. She suggested a healing visualization. Close your eyes and imagine the wound on your chest. Now imagine you are seeing it through a softening lens and quieten it, blur its edges so that it's less disturbing to look at. Now imagine the area being healed by light or words or music or something flowing over it. I imagined looking at the wound through a misty pinkish mauve light, then an emollient cream spreading slowly over my chest. Its creaminess was white, honeyed, soothing. The visualization was very calming. I've tried it again at home and it had the same effect.

I had a good rest in the afternoon and in the evening I ran the Prose and Poetry Workshop. It was good to be teaching again and I didn't flag until the last fifteen minutes. I was nervous about telling the group that I had breast cancer but I knew the news would get round so I was convinced it was best to be direct and open. Of course everyone was very sympathetic.

3rd March

The slightly dizzyish feeling I've had since the operation has gone. I feel strong enough to make appointments to get my hair done and to see the dentist about my broken crown and tooth. Also I've finished the article 'Poets I Go Back To' and I'm just getting into another poem. It's about that first wonderful bath three days after the operation. It needs more material. I'm beginning to miss writing my long narrative poem which I left at the end of January with Section 13 partly drafted. Today too I've started reading some of the poems submitted for an anthology which will show the range and excellence of work by contemporary women poets. It will not confine itself to the trendy, will have a main focus on older poets and will include work by up and coming writers who are little known. One of the original aims of Second Light was to produce such an anthology and Gladys Mary Coles, a poet who also runs Headland Press, agreed to publish the book. Dilys, Gladys Mary and I are co-editors. Dilys and I have also edited a different anthology: *Parents*. The book includes poems by one hundred and fourteen women poets about their own parents.

7th March

I was more tired yesterday and the computer stopped working again last night. I left Ben messages at home and on his mobile phone. He'd been out at the cinema and when he came in he heard me on his answer machine sounding worked up and asking him to ring as soon as possible. 'Who's dead?' he enquired when he returned my call. I told him about the computer. 'Well, your voice sounded as if a major disaster had occurred.' I apologized. It did feel like a disaster to me. 'Mum,' he said as if I was I eight years old, 'I'll always be able to get your computer working quickly if I'm in the country. Computers *do go wrong* and what has happened is not a tragedy.' Feeling ashamed I made supper while he gave Erwin instructions over the phone and within minutes my computer was live again.

I've been feeling anxious for some days as there's been no news from the oncologist about the rest of my results and my follow up treatment. However, he's phoned this evening and he wants me to have some 'gentle chemotherapy' because the cancer had passed through two lymph nodes. The way he spoke it was as if he was offering a lullaby though I'm well aware it won't be that! The first treatment will be on this coming Monday, the next one after our holiday in Nice. I now feel very afraid again, afraid of how the chemotherapy will make me feel, afraid I won't feel well enough to get home afterwards, afraid that the treatment won't stop cancer spreading. It's given by injection and I hate injections. I've been lying in bed terrified that cancer will affect another part of my body in a couple of years in spite of the treatment. I realize I'm extremely ignorant about chemotherapy, that I still associate it with people not getting better even though I now know people who have undergone it and remained well ever since. I know I'm being irrational but the reality of the treatment in a few days makes the illness feel very immediate again.

9th March

I've been very frustrated this morning while trying to find out more about the chemotherapy. However, I've now spoken to a friendly nurse at the clinic who explained they give treatment in cycles, that a cycle consists of two treatments a week apart and that there is then a gap of three weeks before the next cycle. I think I have to go through six of these cycles which sounds awful. Starting this treatment is another

gate to pass through. I can't help feeling worried about how the chemotherapy will affect running my classes and the various fixtures for
readings and courses out of London. I know I must concentrate on the
key issue of making myself safe but I shall be very unhappy if I have to
make cancellations because I want to do my teaching and readings and
I absolutely hate letting people down. Of course Ruth and Mimi keep
reassuring me that everyone will be co-operative and sympathetic.

I didn't record anything else in my notebook about the bath poem
but I remember it came relatively easily. As soon as I started
developing the notes I found myself writing about a kind Irish
nurse who'd helped with the bath and then the last part suddenly
blossomed. Writing this poem was affirming. On March 10th I
was making notes for another poem so I think 'Bath' must have
been finished by March 9th. Here it is:

Bath

Kindness, an Irish lilt in her voice,
spares me the effort of running the water
and supports my elbow when, stripped
of everything but wound dressings,
I take a giant step into the tub.

Warm water wells into my crotch,
unlocks my spine, lullabies my stomach.
Is it because I've passed through
such extremity this comfort is intense
as the yellow which daffodils trumpet?

Yesterday – my raw body stranded
by the basin, chill sprouting on my skin
while a Chinese student nurse
conscientiously dabbed each
helpless area – is miles away.

Dimly, I remember a stark room
and the high-sided saltwater bath
I was dipped in a few days
after giving birth. As Kindness
babies my back with a pink flannel

I'm reborn though maimed, ageing.
And this pool of bliss can no more
be explained than the song that pours
from a lark as it disappears into
stitchless blue, the seed circles

that cram a sunflower's calyx,
day splashing crimsons
and apricot golds across the sky
before it seeps into the silence
of night, the way love fountains.

10th March

I'm still daunted about the number of chemotherapy sessions and I'm on a very short fuse. I'm afraid I've dumped my stress on Erwin. I must discuss this with Kate. I went to see the dentist so that she could examine the damage to my teeth. She said I would need three or four sessions but that it could wait and was very sympathetic. Even so I was exhausted and bothered by the time I got home. I still have nothing like my normal strength.

Some people have the gift of being supportive even though they have problems of their own. Others even though they mean well hit exactly the wrong note. Yesterday I spoke to a friend whom I taught with years ago at a comprehensive school. It was great talking to her at first but then she astonished me by rapping out: 'You'll really regret it if you try and do anything other than a bit of writing for the next few months.' I tried to fend her off by saying I was working out what I could manage as I went along but she went on hectoring me and threw in a few ominous warnings as well. By the time I put the phone down I felt as if I was going to collapse. The conversation was a shock because this friend had always been such a doer of things. Talking it over with Erwin I remembered she had been very ill with blood poisoning a few years ago. 'What you're getting is her agenda, her problems,' he pointed out. I know this must be right but I'm very vulnerable at the moment and her warnings kept me awake last night. I'll cut out whatever I have to, I told myself tearfully, but I also felt angry.

In complete contrast to that phone call is the visit I've just had from Barbara who's in one of my writing groups, a poet with real talent. She turned up with all sorts of herbal tinctures, told me that drinking a lot of water and eating apples would offset the treatment and was full of praise for everything I'm doing. I felt very touched but also guilty that I have been a strain on Erwin. Barbara's mum had cancer for fifteen years. It wasn't discovered early and this was about thirty years ago so there were fewer treatments available. However, she was very much a fighter and used to go round talking to women's groups about coping with cancer.

Shell: Flow-Writing about Georgia O'Keeffe's painting White Shell with Red Hills

A conical shell smooth as a mushroom or a snail shell – the spiral turning itself into a nipple. It is wedded to the body of the red mountain. It wears the mountain's rifts and folds. It offers itself to me. I will pass through its entrance. I will explore its secret corridor, climb its winding stairway soothing as silk. At the top I'll find a tiny aperture, a peephole to the stars. This might be the start of a poem – it needs expanding.

11th March

Shell: Additional note

Shall I grasp this white appendage, ease it off the mountain, mould it to the flatness on my chest so that I'm no longer lopsided? Or shall I approach this (giant beehive?) igloo whose snowy sides will cool the rage in my mind? Shall I enter the sleek building, find it lined with mother-of-pearl?

> I knew this second note had taken the poem further but I think I only had a glimmering that I'd reached its core: rage. I had experienced so much fear since the beginning of the year that I'd not given much thought to the anger simmering beneath the surface and erupting every now and again, mainly in a volley of swear words and angry complaints which poor Erwin couldn't escape even though they weren't usually directed against him.

CHAPTER SIX

First Encounter with Chemotherapy

13th March 2000

The large room I'm sitting in is upstairs in a Georgian house which has high ceilings with elegant plasterwork decoration. The atmosphere is relaxed – there are plenty of easy chairs, a thick carpet and magazines on low tables. All this makes it feel unlike a hospital. The sister in charge of me, who is relaxed and friendly, explained that I'm to be injected with three different chemotherapy drugs and an anti-sickness drug. She also said I could phone the clinic day or night and that they expected – *wanted* – me to phone if I was worried about anything at all. At night I would be put through to the ward where the nurse on duty would be able to see my notes on the computer. I suppose I'd hoped there would be a support system. I'm very relieved that I'm being offered so much help. The pharmacist has also had a talk with me. He's given me Tamoxifen tablets which I'm to start taking today and anti-sickness pills to use at home. 'These,' he said with confidence, holding up the packet, 'are a gold standard. They prevent sickness in 95 per cent of cases.' Gold indeed, I thought, feeling comforted. A breast cancer nurse has been to see me as well and when I told her I was bothered because my arm was still very stiff she said she'd arrange for me to see a physiotherapist.

Middle of the night 13/14th March

Well I've got through the first treatment! I realize my tension had been building up for days beforehand and on Sunday night terror mushroomed in my head. I was afraid I'd be so nauseous that it would be impossible to travel home, that I would be on the point of collapse for hours, days maybe and unable to do anything at all. It was fantastic to come out of the building, see the sky, walk down steps onto a London pavement, find I could walk back to Great Portland Street station and that in spite of feeling drugged I could cope with the tube. Of course it made a big difference that Erwin was with me. When we arrived home there was a message from someone in one of my groups and although I felt muzzy and peculiar it really helped me to phone her back, speak coherently and focus sympathetically on what she wanted to tell me.

I know why I'm awake now. I was told that the cocktail of drugs included a mild steroid and I know steroids have a pep up effect. I react so strongly to medication I'm sure the steroid is preventing me from relaxing. It's not just that I can't sleep, I find it difficult to lie still even. I've now phoned the clinic because my head's aching. The quiet nurse I spoke to was sympathetic but it was clear she thought it was my anxiety that's keeping me awake. It's ironic that the night I felt most worried – last night – I slept with a sleeping pill. It's useless taking a sleeping pill if a drug hypes me up like this so I'm trying to focus on other things.

On Saturday – it seems miles away – Erwin and I went out for lunch and then I did a reading for the Older Feminists' Network. On Sunday we had our N7 workshop – a small group of poet friends which meets in my house something like every six to eight weeks. It was good that the weekend was busy. It helped keep my mind off chemotherapy.

14th March

In spite of not sleeping last night – and I'm still convinced it was because of the steroid – I feel I've passed through another gate. I often have the unpleasant sense of being at the edge of nausea, that medication is only controlling it. However, twice in the night when I felt queasy I felt better as soon as I ate a piece of toast, I tried listening to Kate's tape but it drew too much attention to my body. Relaxing music was better. Around four in the morning I upset a glass of water on the shelf by my bed and it only just missed my notebook. It took me a while to mop up as water had seeped into a couple of paperbacks. The incident, the whole night, began to seem funny. I lay down once more and tried visualizing bands of colour flowing through me. This helped a little. Somewhere around 5a.m. I dozed off.

17th March

On the one hand I'm relieved the experience was no worse – on the other it was still awful. I detest the sense of being invaded by drugs, of being interfered with, turned into something that's not exactly myself. On Tuesday night I slept very deeply but last night wasn't good at all. The best way of managing the day is to do a variety of things in short stints: writing, reading, listening to the radio, talking on the phone. I'm slowly going through poems submitted for the anthology of women's poetry and this reminds me I'm still involved in the outside world. I've also done one or two bits of routine work. The less I think about my body the better. I hate the thought of going through this treatment again. Knowing I am to have radiotherapy as well for a month from the end of April is overwhelming. I'm quite worried about keeping my teaching going. As for my fixtures out of London, I can see some of these will have to go. I feel very tired, sometimes almost at the point of collapse.

> Because the chemotherapy was so much on my mind I'm not surprised that I didn't note anything about writing for several days but I know I must have drafted 'The Shell' at this time. Writing

this poem helped me begin to acknowledge my anger both about the mastectomy and the chemotherapy. Emotionally I couldn't dislodge the sense that I was being maliciously attacked even though I knew intellectually the purpose of the operation and the treatment was to protect me. I use the surreal quite often in writing and Georgia O'Keeffe's painting, which had prompted me into a piece of Flow-Writing on March 10th, offered a safe and in the main metaphorical way to express my anger. The images in the painting were exciting and it felt daring to make use of them. I remember I had trouble with the first verse of the poem but the rest came quite quickly and I did no more than tidy it up afterwards. Here is the final version:

The Shell

is smooth as a white mushroom cap,
conical, married to the rifts and curves
of a hill's geranium flank, and its spiral
soon culminates in a satisfying nipple.

Shall I scoop up this shell, go
down to the field where no sheep
graze, plant it on the forlorn flesh,
pretend my chest's refound its shape?

Better to recognize the protuberance
is large as an igloo, hug the side
to soothe my wound, its flood tide
of anger redder than rosebuds

than the mountain's pelt, than my blood.
Once I've found a way inside
I'll ignore the mother-of-pearl wall,
hurry down the corridor, climb all

the stairs, break the silken silence
as I bore a hole in the roof, untie
my coiled rage, let it erupt,
fan into flames that sweep the sky.

19th March

Note/Flow-Writing about Georgia O'Keeffe's painting
The White Iris

I have crossed into another country, do not know where I am standing, even if I am able to stand. How to approach the extraordinary territory before me. The great white slopes are beautifully moulded but I don't know what kind of earth or if any earth lies beneath them. If I attempt to climb will this beautiful white hill, its straight furrow, take my weight? I am no longer sure what weight I have and I fear I can't attempt the final steep ascent to the crest much as I long to visit it, to discover what its crown of gold and lemon flames are – no, not flames because although the glow is intense there is no suggestion of flickering fire. The lemon segments of the flowers, which make up the landscape, pull me towards them and yet I am terrified of this hypnotic place, of losing control. Over the rim of the crest steeper mountains or clouds are melting into a sky alight with the sun's wings. This is a window to an elsewhere.

> Looking at this piece of writing now I remember what a release it was to write about my fear of chemotherapy through the painting, to allow myself to see a landscape in the flower and then follow my flow of thoughts and images. I didn't plan to use the

painting in this way. Both *The White Iris* and *White Shell with Red Hills* are reproductions in a small book I have of Georgia O'Keeffe's paintings. It was almost as if they were waiting for me. Oddly enough a few months previously I had looked through the book thinking I'm sure some of these could be starting points for poems but when I tried to pick one to write about nothing clicked.

20th March

At the clinic while waiting for the next dose of chemotherapy

Yesterday morning I spoke to John who was very calm and reassuring about the course we're supposed to be running together at the end of next month at Holland House in Worcestershire. Luckily Kate Foley, a good poet who's published two books, is coming on the course and she's already agreed to give some help. John said it wouldn't be any problem at all if he runs the course with Kate. He also said he liked 'Bath'. He only received it a few days ago because his computer had been out of action. I read 'Shell' to him over the phone and he was very positive about it but of course he needs to see it written down. I told him how buoyed up I am that 'Today There Is Time' and 'Snowdrops' have been accepted by the journal *Scintilla*. His comment was: 'Don't ever tell me again that you have difficulties in getting poems published.'

In the afternoon Erwin and I went to Trent Park. The grounds of the house and the rolling land with woods and farms round it is our nearest piece of countryside and it only takes ten minutes or so to drive there. It was full of families and dogs and it was beautiful with its new green layers of willows, the light glittering on the lakes, bushes budding on the slopes. In the watergarden I saw scatterings of my childhood flowers: celandine, primroses and wood anemones. Daffodils were growing everywhere and the pools were gun metal green. I felt a special enjoyment in everything.

24th March

At the clinic on Monday I stressed – thanks to Dilys urging me to report it – how hyper the steroid had made me. The oncologist decided not to include it with my treatment this time. I was a bit apprehensive in case I suffered some adverse effects as the steroid is supposed to help the anti-emetic drugs move round my system. However, I've come through much better, slept better and I didn't feel nearly so hyped up. Nevertheless it's been difficult to focus even for a short time on any work requiring concentration. By Wednesday I felt rather better and yesterday I had a sense of the whole thing lifting. However, on Wednesday night my gums were stinging and they bled as soon as I touched them with my toothbrush. I phoned the clinic yesterday morning and the nurse I spoke to said: ' I'd like you to come in so that I can make sure you're all right.' I was impressed by the care being taken. Also there was something exhilarating about making the phone call at 9.50a.m., getting dressed and out of the house in half an hour, sitting on the tube drafting 'Elsewhere' – which has grown out of the *White Iris* notes – and finding myself in the clinic drinking coffee by 10.50. My mouth was examined and I was told to use a child's toothbrush and toothpaste, also to use the mouthwash Corsodyl diluted. My gums are already less sore. Today though I feel worn out. We met Ruth and Michael for a snack lunch. It was supposed to be a treat but the place was busy with business people having lunch and they were not only slow in bringing the food but made a mistake with the order which I found extremely irritating. I realize I need to relax more, not force anything.

26th March

A gift of this illness is that it has given me 'time'. I've felt short of time for years, was always planning how to fit things in. Now, because I'm limited in what I can do, I can take time for all sorts of little things, play with time. I'm relieved I've left Flightways – it's one less thing to worry about although I am sure, once I'm better, I am going to miss working there every Monday, miss especially Abdul and the other people I've been teaching – some of them for years. However, I'm now very aware I must choose essentials and give myself space. Sometimes it is good just to enjoy being still – the sensation of stillness. Just now I am looking at the frost in the park and garden, the brightness of the Easter rose, its orange flowers not quite open. There is a blue tit on the clothes-line, maybe searching for insects. On the fence is a robin but there are no sparrows about. There used to be so many chirping near the house. One usually made a nest in the flue from the defunct boiler. Our newspaper is always printing articles offering reasons as to why they've disappeared from London streets and suburbs.

28th March

When I spoke to John on Sunday he said 'Elsewhere' worked. Because of its surreal character I was very unsure how it would come over. Of course it could apply to other illnesses, ordeals:

Elsewhere

How to approach this territory?
The slopes are beautifully sculpted
but are they based on rock layers
or a vacuum which will suck me in?
Even if the magnolia surface can bear
my weight I've no reason to suppose
I can remain queen of my legs.

There is no choice. Terrified,
I start to climb, know at once
potent invaders are racing through
my channels, taking me over. Appalled,
my inner systems signal rebellion.
What resources can I muster
to contain the battle in my body?

Somehow I must manage the ascent
to the crest with its glowing crown
of gold and lemon crescents which lie
like poised tongues, then pass through
the opening within the ring of peaks
and move beyond elsewhere to meet
snow-white clouds banked with possibility.

Kate gave me a massage yesterday afternoon – she offers therapeutic massage as well as psychotherapy. She was very gentle. I was aware of my body as fragile and tensed from its ordeal, of it beginning to unwind. In the evening I managed to run my seminar. This group, for four poets committed to developing their work, is intensive. The session went well but I became very tired towards the end of it. I felt rather better afterwards when I didn't have to concentrate any more. In general if I get tired I seem to pick up quite quickly if I take a complete break – maybe lie down and listen to relaxing music.

My perception of the marathon of chemotherapy – what I'll be able to do during the treatment – is changing all the time. As my energy continues to be very low I've found myself wondering if it's unrealistic to consider doing any out of London engagements at all for the next few months. I suspect I'll have to cancel everything except the reading to Suffolk Poetry Society which is at a venue near Ipswich – quite a short journey. I'll note how I pick up from this cycle of chemotherapy. I've certainly been weakened by it so I'd better be ready to cancel things. I found myself crying when I lay down after lunch. Everything felt too much and as if I'll never get out of the tunnel of treatment. After I'd had a good moan to Ruth on the phone I began to 'rise again' – enough to enjoy the normality of going to Palmers Green and buying red slippers which I badly need as the old ones are worn right through.

29th March

This morning on the train on the way up to the clinic for a blood test at what they call the low point in the cycle I started drafting 'Words' – part Fourteen of my long narrative poem. After the diagnosis it was impossible to think about it again until last week. I'd already produced some notes in January but I thought it would be very difficult getting back into the poem again. This next section is in rhyme too. However, I'm surprised and pleased by the progress I'm making. I think the 'cancer' sequence needs a 'down' poem if I can think of a way of writing one. Would another painting be a starting point?

1st April

Erwin's birthday today. We went out for a meal. It was fun and I'm glad we've had some kind of celebration. My sleep is still badly disrupted by the chemotherapy and this is making life very hard. I don't know if the Tamoxifen plays a part in this. I keep waking up during the night needing to go to the loo and usually feeling a bit queasy. Eating a biscuit and drinking water helps but once awake it's hard to get back to sleep and my anxiety grows. In spite of everything the 'Words' section is moving on and my ideas for the next few sections are clarifying.

5th April

Image Exploration: 'The Cave'

It is darkish and dank. The damp, which seems to grow in the cave walls, the ground, the air above, is chilling. It's eating into my body. I feel less than myself, lost, without any bearings, cut off. I can make out passageways ahead of me, each leading into a darkness more profound than anything I have ever known, ever imagined. This could be the underworld, the kingdom of death. I have been closer to death than I wanted to be and here I can smell its clammy breath, the breath of a mountainous dog greedy to consume me. I do not want to die. I want to find life again, a chink in all the ridged and jagged layers above me, a route to dry air and colour and sky. I can make out stalactites – they reach from the roof almost to the floor of the cave – and also a mean army of skeletons waiting to attack. Drip drip drip – water trickling – everything wet. I have a terrible sense that there is no way out, that the passages ahead only lead further in.

An echoing sound, a calling, gonging sound, not loud but eerie. It seems to be coming closer. I want contact but not with that inhuman sound. But is it inhuman? Now it seems to be more like a wailing, a lamentation, to be uttering something of the shape of words – or am I delirious in my fear? 'W-where a-are you-ou?' almost owl-like. The voice is distorted as if speaking down a pipe and yet isn't it my father? Do I want to find him? I've spoken to him in my writing. Why has he turned up again and in this form?

I turn round, resolutely I turn my back on the voice. And now I can hear it much more distinctly, its anger rising. 'Come here, now you've come this far. Explain yourself and your actions.'

'No,' I say, 'I've grown beyond you. I have my own life now.'

His laugh is mocking: 'Some life. You've been ill, you've been lopped and maimed. You've had what you deserved.'

'No,' I scream. 'I've made something of my life and I've moved beyond you and I've made something of my illness.' Am I imagining it or is it lighter ahead? I slip on a flat stone but I'm soon on my feet. It's a struggle but I go on towards the pale light. Sky, I can see sky. The passage broadens. I stumble out onto a hillside mauve with ling heather.

I wrote this piece in my notebook during my Prose and Poetry Workshop. It happened that almost all the group were away because of illness, holidays or work commitments. Of the two who came one had brought a long short story. Before we looked at that in detail we had time for a substantial writing exercise and I decided we'd try out the 'The Cave' Image Exploration which I'd planned for the 'Inner and Outer Landscapes' course at Holland House at the end of the month. (This exercise is included in Image Exploration 1. in the 'Writing Ideas' section of this book.)

I was surprised and moved by what I wrote. I hadn't expected my dominating father, who was no longer alive, to have any connection with my illness. And yet more than once I'd heard a critical voice in my head saying: 'It's your fault you're ill.' I don't usually read out what I write in workshops but I did so on this occasion and the other two, who'd written striking pieces themselves, were impressed by the force of feeling I'd expressed. I realized it wasn't chance I'd thought up the cave image as a starting point and I knew the piece was something I'd come back to.

6th April

Anna Adams phoned up. I've known Anna since around 1984. She's a well-respected poet who deserves to be better known. She had a heart operation last year and I was pleased to hear that she was making a good recovery from it. After we'd been talking for a while it dawned on me that she knew nothing about my illness and that I was going to have to tell her over the phone. 'Take a deep breath, Anna,' I said when she asked me how I was. I took a deep breath myself. However, it turned out she'd had a mastectomy about forty years ago when her children were aged four and two. She said there were secondaries but chemotherapy was not available in Britain at that time and explained: 'My father wanted to pay with money he hadn't got to send me to the States for this new treatment but I didn't feel I could leave the children.' She was given radiotherapy which was very much cruder than it is now. She's not had any recurrence. She said the whole thing affected her psychologically and that it was because of the illness that she started writing much more seriously. I found the conversation uplifting.

Of course it's amazing that modern medicine has so many techniques but every now and then I have a bad moment when I think about all the bits of my body I've lost: my womb, one ovary, a breast, as well as a lens in my right eye. But my right eye sees wonderfully now with an artificial lens.

It's suddenly hit me that I've tumbled on the material for a 'down' poem: 'The Cave'.

Note for 'The Cave'

Damp clinging weight of rocks, the chill eating greedily into me, a rank smell. The voice of the father pursuing, the voice of punishment, and – this is important – my turning away after I've spoken to him and reaching that hill covered with heather.

CHAPTER SEVEN

Interlude in Nice

8th April 2000

We're in Nice! Ten days ago I felt so weak I couldn't even imagine making the journey to the airport and I phoned the clinic to query whether I would be strong enough to travel. I hadn't realized the chemotherapy would continue to make me feel weak afterwards. The nurse I spoke to was reassuring and I've made it – I'm *so* pleased. We arrived yesterday and it's wonderful to be somewhere so different, so away from the state of illness. I love the blues of the sea; the palms everywhere, their trunks cross-hatched like pineapples; the air of luxury; the gardens with fountains; the hills behind the town; the globe lamps of the street lighting; all the restaurants and cafés. And it's lovely to sit outside or half outside and watch the world going by.

Today we went to the Matisse Museum where we saw some of his famous blue cut-outs in which the female body is turned into a series of silhouette patterns with head, arm, breast, knee, leg sharply and deftly defined and with a subtle change of position in each image. Of course I noticed how much the figures are characterized by their breasts.

9th April

'The Cave': Notes

My mind is at work to turn this into a poem. I know the father part is central. Inside me I heard him speaking these words: 'You have lost your womb, an ovary, a breast – not much left of you, not much of a woman, are you?' These details presented themselves too: a sense of collapse, whirr of wings, bats rushing for my eyes. A sense of the inimitable blues of the Mediterranean Sea. I turn, stumble away, away from his voice. A small round eye of light in the distance. It widens. Suddenly I'm spilled onto a hillside and there's the sweetness of pink bell heather, a sky blue as a forget-me-not.

14th April

I'm writing this on the plane. I'm glad we kept the Chagall Museum for yesterday, the last day, because that was the jewel of all the jewels in the crown! My first impression was of colour jumping from the walls, its intensity and generosity. In the huge central hall and in the other rooms too, each painting has been given the space it really needs and there are plenty of benches to sit on so the gallery is easy to visit. Almost all the paintings have a biblical theme. The central hall is stunning with huge canvasses of figures from the early books of the Old Testament including Jacob, silver light on his braced legs as he struggles with the angel; Abraham dramatically poised; Noah sleeping on the grass after the flood has receded.

We were sitting down quite soon after we arrived when I became aware of a girl aged about nine who was sharing our bench. She was leaning over sheets of paper and I suddenly saw she was reading Braille. I found it distressing that a blind child had been brought into this world of colour. After a little she went off with a slight, attractive and very chic woman. I saw the child's eyes were half closed and looked sore. She remained in my mind as we went to the concert hall to look at the stained glass windows depicting the creation and as we feasted in other rooms. Later when we were gazing at Adam and Eve in paradise the little girl was brought to the painting and placed within inches of a wolf at the bottom of the canvas. It dawned on me that she had peripheral vision and I was very moved that she could in fact see something. After a minute or two she turned abruptly and was led away. Her image haunted me for the rest of the day.

> Afterwards I knew I wanted to write a poem about the blind girl and she came into my mind several times during the summer but it was September before I attempted a poem and when I did I found it very problematic.

In the afternoon we had tea and afterwards we sat by the sea for half an hour. I love the Mediterranean's different tones – light blue close to the shore, deep blue further out. The water was rough and great waves broke on the beach.

This has been a fantastic holiday, one of the best we've ever had. I think I'd have felt that anyway but escaping from illness and treatment has made it even more special. My energy has held up much better than I expected and although I've felt queasy at times this has been progressively less often. I'm worried though that the chemotherapy will have an accumulative effect. A few days ago I was dismayed when quite a lot of hair came away on my hairbrush. But I'm telling myself that all I've done and seen this week will help to sustain me during the next few months.

CHAPTER EIGHT

Chemotherapy and Radiotherapy 1

19th April 2000

I felt a big dip when we came home on Saturday. I nearly always feel disorientated after holidays but this was much worse. I suppose it's because my strength is still limited and because I now have to face months of treatment. It didn't help that the weather was cold, grey and rainy. On Sunday I felt better and much more able to take in that *Scintilla* has now accepted 'Bath', 'The Shell' and 'Elsewhere' as well as 'Today There Is Time' and 'Snowdrops'. I've now formally put the poems together as a sequence which I've titled *Repair*. The reference is to the last line of 'Today There Is Time'. This is the theme of all the poems – and I still feel that strong connection with C.K. Williams' *Repair*.

Scintilla, the journal of the Usk Valley Vaughan Association, comes out once a year. It publishes essays which have a direct or indirect connection with the metaphysical poet, Henry Vaughan, and his twin brother, Thomas Vaughan. It also includes new poetry which has a spiritual dimension. I've been in touch with Anne Cluysenaar, who is one of the editors, for about three years and we've become friends over the phone. Anne lives on a smallholding near Usk and her own poetry, which expresses an affinity with nature, explores deeply both the spiritual and intellectual. Anne and I finally met in March because she was in London to do a reading and came over to see me the day after my second chemotherapy treatment. It was strange to meet someone for the first time when I was so below par, so not myself, but it was easy and enjoyable as Anne has a warm manner and talks with such enthusiasm and knowledge on many subjects. It was when she visited that she asked to see the cancer poems so I sent her the first two and later on the others as she was so responsive.

On Monday Erwin and I agreed there was no need for him to come to the clinic until lunchtime. As I walked to the tube station I was aware of feeling much stronger physically than I did five weeks ago. Soon after I arrived I asked one of the nurses how long it takes to recover after all the chemotherapy treatments are finished. I was very shaken when she told me that some doctors say it takes six months and also that the effects might intensify as treatment proceeds. The next day I spoke to Mary MacRae whom I've been getting to know since October. Mary had a mastectomy followed by chemotherapy last year and she said I would have reasonable strength after a few weeks but I still felt very cast down for a while on Monday morning.

Almost as soon as I'd had the routine blood test I went down to the basement for a preparatory session for the radiotherapy. The radiotherapists make careful measurements and calculations so that the treatment is given to a very exact area of the body. Despite this I found the session stressful as I had to lie for something like forty-five minutes in the same position with my hands clasped behind my head. This became more and more uncomfortable as time went on. Tears came into my eyes and I felt very upset about facing the next few months. Nice and all those paintings I'd looked at seemed far, far away – an illusion. However, things brightened up later when Erwin arrived with a letter that had come in the second post. It was from Peter Sansom, the editor of the *North* magazine, saying the 'Poets I Go Back To' article was just right and also that he was interested in publishing 'I'm Not

Going To Tell Her' if I made a few changes. I actually managed to revise the poem during the chemotherapy by using my left hand as the other was trapped – attached to tubes feeding in drugs and water. Concentrating on the poem enabled me to separate myself from the treatment and all this lifted me from the trough I'd sunk into during the morning.

When I arrived home I was rather more focused than after the last session but I also felt somewhat queasier. I made a start on the proofs of my new and selected poems, *Insisting on Yellow*, which had arrived in the morning's first post. It was such a boost to go through these and think of the book being launched in October when all this horrible treatment would be behind me. Because I was drugged I only allowed myself to look at a few pages, braced myself to concentrate fully. Each line I read felt like a thrust against cancer. I'm continuing to read the poems in short stints. There aren't many errors – the occasional letter missing at the end of a word, a mistake in a title, nothing drastic.

I am dreading the mix of chemotherapy and radiotherapy in the second half of May. I must look at ways of making life as easy as possible during that time. Today I had a second session of preparation for radiotherapy. This was also uncomfortable for my arm but it wasn't as long as the session on Monday and I managed to cut myself off from the last few minutes by going through Kate's 'Egg of Protection' visualization. I've finally managed to get the 'Words' section of the long narrative poem onto the computer. I've also word-processed the image exploration and my later notes about 'The Cave'. Everything tells me this is material for a key poem.

23rd April

Yesterday was a very distressing day. I came in from a short walk to find Mimi had left a message on my phone saying she had sad news about Colin which she didn't want to leave on the answerphone. Colin – a close poet friend – has been suffering from a serious mental illness for four years which was eventually identified as manic depression but for the last three months he'd shown signs of being very much better.

From Mimi's tone I was immediately certain he was no longer alive. At the verge of tears and trembling I dialled her number and she told me Colin had been found dead and that it was almost certain he'd collapsed from a heart attack. Only a few weeks ago I had an extremely positive conversation with him on the phone. He'd been much less bound up with himself, talking about books and poetry again and he was very sympathetic about my illness. He said he'd put a new manuscript together and he spoke both enthusiastically and realistically about it. He also told me about the computer course he'd done at Mind, an organization which supports people who have mental health problems, and their interest in using him to teach computing. In fact for the first time since his breakdown he sounded like the pre-illness Colin. Now this. He was only fifty.

In the afternoon I had a long talk with Colin's wife, Maggie, whom I'm very fond of. She was amazingly composed, perhaps because she needed to be to support their two daughters. She's been put under enormous strain by his depression and manic behaviour and although, as she said, she had in a sense lost him four years ago, they'd had a close relationship and she was still very fond of him. We talked about the fact that Colin hadn't been in very good physical shape as he smoked heavily and often stayed up all night. She also said she was very grateful for the last few weeks when he'd been much more like himself and they'd become much closer again.

I felt shaken all day. Colin was my first writing friend. We met at a writing group – in 1982, I think – and for about two years we commented in detail by post on one another's work. He was brilliantly clever, had an almost photographic memory and strong views about writers. His first collection of poetry received good notices including one in *Poetry Review*. The second, which was in parts obscure, passed almost unnoticed and his illness took him further away from public notice. Although a few people knew what a good writer he was his work hasn't had anything like the attention it deserved. John was upset to hear about Colin when I talked to him this morning. As Editor of the Littlewood Press he'd published Colin's first book in 1987 so he'd had quite a lot of contact with him. John and I agreed at once that we should edit Colin's new manuscript and find a way of getting it published.

25th April

I've been making up visualizations to 'help' my white corpuscles – it's a therapeutic game. While I'm lying in bed or in other spare moments, with my eyes closed, I say inwardly: 'White corpuscles up up – any stray cancer cells down down.' And I picture the white corpuscles as small golden gondolas nosing their way down the Grand Canal in Venice, under the Rialto bridge, out to the wider waterways. I begin to picture the great churches: St. Mark's, Santa Maria della Salute, St. Giorgio Maggiore and Redentore. I've also pictured the white corpuscles as ballet dancers on stage, the swans in *Swan Lake* standing on their points, legs rising, their every movement kicking down any seed of cancer. I expect I'll think up some more images.

Today is the beginning of the marathon of radiotherapy. I am worried about the damage it will do to me and find it difficult to 'feel' that the treatment will be beneficial. I have to make twenty-five visits to Harley Street – every day except for weekends. Twenty-five times of getting off the tube at Warren Street or Great Portland Street and trudging to the clinic, lying under the monstrous machine for a few minutes and then trudging back.

All the time I am becoming more adept at doing things in small stints and I am making use of things like glucose tablets – Dilys' idea – when I go for treatment and at other tiring times. I also make sure I take water with me whenever I go out and something easy to eat like fig rolls or a banana. I cope with food best by eating small amounts quite often. The digestive biscuits which I munch when I wake in the middle of the night I now keep by the bed and I always have phone conversations propped up in bed so that I am physically resting. The routine of having breakfast when I wake, then doing some writing, then lying in bed often thinking about writing before going onto something else or occasionally back to writing, works well. I get dressed, which is somehow very tiring, towards the end of the morning and do my arm exercises before lunch.

I thought about Colin a lot over the weekend and felt sad. On Sunday our writing group met and I was so pleased to see Caroline again. She spent an afternoon with me in February. John introduced us in 1986, a year or so before he published her first collection of poetry which was launched in Highgate with Colin's first book, and we've been close friends ever since. She's a violinist and teaches music. Because she lives in Tunbridge Wells we usually meet in central London and have several hours together two or three times a year, talking about anything and everything, looking at one another's poems and sometimes going to an art gallery. It so happened we met on January 5th, the day I received the letter calling me back to the hospital following my breast screening. She was very sympathetic and has kept in close touch during this time.

Colin, Caroline and I started our Sunday workshops soon after I got to know Caroline because we didn't find other larger groups sufficiently helpful and we were keen to work in depth with a few people really committed to developing their writing. It seems a strange coincidence that the group had a session two days after Colin's death. I'd phoned Caroline to give her the news on Friday and of course we talked a lot about Colin in the meeting. During his illness he attended erratically and about a year and a half ago he turned up in a very manic state, unable to focus, but he came again this January with two very poignant poems about people on the mental health ward. It's good to have that memory of him.

2nd May

Soon after our holiday I had finally acknowledged that I wouldn't be strong enough to go to Worcestershire on April 28th and co-run the writing course I'd organized. It was a great relief to know that Kate Foley was going to stand in for me and she helped to make the weekend a great success. John enjoyed working with her and I received three e-mails immediately afterwards from people saying how brilliant it was. This was uplifting – and touching as they also said that I was missed! John said he was excited by the high standard of the writing and he has booked for us to run another course next May. I was also touched that Kate said she wanted to come back next year as a student. This year the subject was inner and outer landscapes. We need a new topic for next year.

Although I'm engaged with other things I often feel panicky about the second half of this month when I will have to undergo two chemotherapy sessions in the later part of the radiotherapy course. By then I wonder how I will be feeling – I've been told the radiotherapy has a cumulative effect of tiredness. I'm trying to keep calm, telling myself to expect very little of the next few months and to regard everything I do as an achievement, rather than fretting about what I can't do. I'd like to build in listening to one side of the relaxation tape every day. At times I feel sunk under as if I will never escape from the trap of weakness.

I have written 'The Cave' and I am amazed at the way it fits into *The Repair* sequence as the hillside at the end relates to the hill in 'The Shell' which I am placing before it and to the slopes in 'Elsewhere' which comes after it. I feel the sequence is incomplete without it. John thinks the poem is powerful but he said the final details seemed too gentle and that something sharper was needed. I saw at once he was right and it didn't take me very long to make the end stronger.

The Cave

Rocks wall me in. Their turbulent layers
jammed together press unbearably
on my head. The clammy air spawns
moisture beads on ledges, ridges,
trickles down long stone faces.
Feeble light and the passages ahead
offer a darkness more profound
than anything I've ever known, imagined.

Stalagmites reach from floor to roof,
a mean band of skeletons waiting
to embrace me. An owl call becomes
a human voice lengthened as if
it had travelled down a pipe: the father
I thought I'd escaped. His hollow sentences
swell, resound on the cave walls:
It's your own fault you're so fallen –

if you'd stayed in your inconspicuous place
you'd not be wombless now, not be one-
breasted, hardly a woman. The words
rush at me: huge-winged birds
greedy to tear and gobble. Nowhere
to retreat. In a moment my sad flesh
will be stabbed, my bones broken.
But a small *no* begins to form

in my head. It holds the inimitable blues
of the Mediterranean Sea and I manage
to cry: *I've become a deeper me.* Slowly
I back from the final judgement, body
flat to the rockside. At last I spy the eye
of day, am spewed onto a hillside,
feel the rough sweetness of bell heather,
the bright sky beginning to heal me.

I've already corrected proofs for *Scintilla* but I mentioned to Anne over
the phone how sorry I was that it was too late to offer her 'The Cave'.
She asked me to send it to her at once and came back to me very

quickly saying how much she liked it. To my surprise she also said it might be possible to include it because there was some unexpected space. I'd be really pleased if she could. I have the sense of these poems being lifted from my hands for publication as I finish them. It's extraordinary. Anne's belief in these poems and her wish to publish them has been amazing.

8th May

I'm very encouraged by the response I've received from Caroline to 'Letter' and 'Words', the two new sections of my long narrative poem. I gave these to her at the last Sunday workshop. She suggested some sharp pruning in one part of the 'Letter' section and also some clarification as she was confused at one point.

9th May

Cancer and jam, cancer and anger.
The anger keeps oozing out like pus, breaking out like a rash.
I'm angry if I drop something.
I'm angry because I keep losing my glasses.
I'm angry because the skin of my fingers is sore from chemotherapy.
I'm angry because my life's been interrupted.
I'm angry because I'm pushed on one side.
I'm angry because I can't do what I want to.
I'm angry because my body's been invaded by treatments.
I'm angry with the nurses, the specialist, everyone at the clinic even though I know their intention is to help me.
I'm angry because the drugs make me feel queasy and weak-legged.
I'm angry because I'm unable to eat much at a time.
I'm angry because I can't do much at a time.
I'm angry because I'm afraid I'll never have a full life again.
I'm angry because I wake up four times every night.
I'm angry because the overpowering sickly sweet smell of the air-freshener in the loo at the clinic makes me feel nauseated.

I'm angry because I'm missing out.
I'm angry because the treatment goes on over so many months.
I'm angry because I'm hot.
I'm angry because I'm cold.
I'm angry because I have to keep considering other people's anxieties.
I'm angry because some people's help is misplaced and unhelpful.
I'm angry because other awful things have happened.

Notes for 'Angry' poem

What does it feel like, this anger? What does it smell of? What does it sound like? It is bubbling in my body like a mob of prisoners. I want to throw it out, slap it like the sea on the shore. I shall shove it out like a bin of rubbish. I want to hit it into faces, wave it from steeples, dangle it in red flags from the thousand windows of a great glass building. Crash! I'll crash it against walls, kick it along pavements, throw out its slops. I am going to make a great scene about it, a drama that will shock audiences into silence, scribble it in furious red across the clean page of the sky, smash bottlefuls of it on the pavement by Warren Street tube station...

I think this will make a 'List' poem if I build up the scale and the extravagance. Writing all this has been a breakthrough. It feels as if – well I am – taking energetic action with my anger and it's incredibly releasing, exciting, fun!

CHAPTER NINE

Chemotherapy and Radiotherapy 2

15th May 2000

I'm starting this entry on the train on my way up for chemotherapy and I'll continue with it while I'm waiting for the treatment. The last time I saw the oncologist I told him I had little energy and he recommended something called noni juice as a food supplement. To my surprise I found this on my way back to the tube in an Indian health and food shop in Warren Street. I almost laughed out loud when a huge dark bottle was placed on the counter. Noni is a small brown Polynesian fruit which, according to the bottle's label and the website, has been used for health reasons in Polynesia, Asia and Hawaii for over two thousand years. It's supposed to attack cancer cells. It was very expensive and I was offered two bottles with £10 off which I agreed to. Because they were so heavy I had to arrange to take them home one at a time. I've definitely felt a bit better this last week. Is this because I'm further away from the chemo treatment or is it the effect of the noni juice which tastes foul even with its added grape juice? My life has been restricted with the daily grind of going up to Harley Street to lie under that mighty machine. I separate myself from the two half minutes of treatment by visualizing a beautiful colour or by counting. The girls who manage the machines are always very pleasant and during the tube journey I've written in my notebook or read. Nevertheless the whole thing is a drag and almost from the first session I felt a burning afterwards on my skin which is very sensitive.

Last week I broke out a bit. On Tuesday I had the radiotherapy quite late and then met Dilys at the Cavendish Hotel in Jermyn Street where I really enjoyed a smoked salmon supper and talking to her before going to the launch of Mimi's *Selected Poems* at Waterstone's in Piccadilly – the first big event I've been to since my operation. Mimi's doing a residency for the Royal Mail and they sponsored the evening. The large room at the top of the shop was packed and there were several notables in the audience. Although she's well-known, her work is not fully appreciated and some critics describe her writing as exotic and Persian without reading properly and ignoring the fact that she's spent most of her life in England. Mimi was wearing a glitzy top. She read beautifully and chose poems which showed the range of her writing including a group from *Entries on Light*, her last book. I love this sequence. I managed to stay until the end of the formal part of the launch by which time I felt very tired. I talked to many people I know and several of them said I looked well (which I found a bit surprising but naturally the comments made me feel better!) and I was touched by everyone's sympathy. I walked to the tube feeling a bit weak but elated by Mimi's poems and the enthusiasm for her.

Just before the evening began I spoke for a moment to Les Murray who's over here from Australia doing a reading tour. Les has been extraordinarily supportive of my writing for several years. As well as being a world famous poet he's the Literary Editor of *Quadrant*, a leading cultural journal in Australia. Over the last few years I think he must have published about twenty-five of my poems. He writes an extremely lively and interesting letter and we correspond occasionally. I hadn't been in touch with him for several months and he knew nothing about my illness. He was seriously ill himself a couple of years ago and I found it very awkward telling him what had happened to me. I could see he was shaken. I'm going to write to him soon and send him some of the cancer poems.

Going out and doing something different gave me such a lift that Erwin and I went to the cinema on Thursday after the radiotherapy session. On Saturday we made the most of the time furthest away from the chemo and went to the theatre for the first time since my operation to see *Cressida*. Yesterday evening Ben and Pogle came to see us and Ben cooked a splendid supper: sea bass, rice and asparagus. He brought his own frying pan – I have nothing that he considers good enough! Ruth and Michael were also invited to savour his cooking which was much appreciated and it was a very enjoyable, chatty evening.

I've had a lovely letter from Grevel Lindop. We met when we did a reading together several years ago in Norwich. His poetry is both thoughtful and approachable. Often his writing is celebratory but it's sharp and poignant too. He's in the process of giving up being a professor at Manchester University in order to write full time and we keep in touch with occasional letters and even more occasional meetings. His *Selected Poems* were published recently so I've dipped into his poetry again and a week or so ago I sent him a note about the book. I also told him about my illness and how writing had supported me. His reply was extraordinarily understanding. He said it was wonderful that writing had helped me, that my letter confirmed his belief in its power. He also mentioned that he would like to do some readings in London to publicize his new book and asked if I had any ideas.

I've spoken to the organizer of the weekly readings the Poetry School puts on at the Poetry Café in Covent Garden and she agreed at once that Grevel should be offered a reading. When I phoned him up to tell him he was amazed I'd responded immediately. I said doing so made me feel I could take action even though I was physically weak. He talked again with great insight about writing giving me support. He'd been intending to give me his *Selected Poems* as a present but as I'd bought it he sent me *The Path & The Palace*, two published lectures on the nature of poetry.

16th May

Yesterday was a day I'd been dreading and it turned out to be very long and uncomfortable. It did help a bit that my radiotherapy session was brought forward to the morning otherwise I'd have had to stay on for it after the chemo treatment. There was a particularly long wait for this and I was extremely tired, thick in the head and queasy by the time we got home. Still I managed to write a note to Irene, Colin's mother. I'd met her at the launches of Colin's books and she's sent me a card because Maggie told her about my illness and also about the intention to produce a book of Colin's poetry. She sweetly wished me better. Understandably she needed to voice her distress about Colin's death. She talked about the new collection and I was glad that the book was something positive for her to hold onto. Neither she nor her husband are at all well and I feel such sympathy for them. Focusing on writing a note to Irene removed me from myself and how awful I felt, transformed it somehow into doing something worthwhile. I used a card which has a Chinese character as its design. I feel there is something calm and timeless about it.

It's very encouraging that the narrative poem is moving on. I've now drafted 'The Ladder' which is part seventeen so in the last few weeks I've completed one section and added three more. I've continued to look at poems for the anthology of women's poetry and in connection with this I've been re-reading one or two collections. I like having this project to concentrate on as it takes me far away from weakness and dragging myself up to the centre of London each day for the wretched radiotherapy.

18th May

I've drafted the anger poem and am calling it 'Release' because that's what it is – a fantastic release to give myself permission to let my feelings out instead of holding them in and trying to be reasonable. It was so satisfying to spend time wallowing in anger and such fun finding increasingly extravagant images for it. It felt as if I actually was kicking anger about, chucking it, hurling it and it's extraordinary how much better I feel for writing the poem. I wasn't sure how John would react to it but he was extremely enthusiastic.

Release

I'm going to slap my anger onto a wet slab,
 put it through a mangle,
hang out its long line of eccentric washing.
 I'm going to fly its flags
from my windows, smack it into surprised faces,
 push it up noses,
smash green bottles of it to smithereens
 on pavements, daub its shout
over walls, hurl it down a football field,
 kick it into goal,
empty it into a dustcart's masticating jaws.

 I'll parade my anger through
town centres, exhibit it in galleries, make
 such a production of it
on stages that audiences will be pinned
 to shocked silence. I'm going
to drive it up the motorway in a topless car,
 scatter its pungent seeds
on ploughed fields, wait for the dark fruits
 to ripen. Then I'll celebrate by
scribbling indelible berry juice across
 the clean page of the sky.

19th May

I had a dreadful journey to the clinic yesterday. There was a hold up on the Piccadilly Line and forty minutes after Erwin dropped me at Arnos Grove Station I had only travelled two stops to Wood Green. Here we were advised to use other means of transport because the station manager could not say when the service would be resumed. Feeling hot, weak and worried I went up to ground level and phoned Erwin who, probably because he was having a rest, didn't answer. I left him a panicky message telling him to warn the clinic I would be late.

Continuity is important in this treatment so I knew I must get myself there however late I was. I wanted to take a taxi to Finsbury Park where I could pick up the Victoria Line but there was no taxi to be seen anywhere so I climbed onto a bus which ground its slow way through Wood Green's traffic-packed shopping centre and on up busy Green Lanes stopping every few yards for what seemed like hours. The sun, which has not been in evidence much lately, shone fiercely as we clanked along. Sweaty and helpless I watched the minutes going by on my watch as I inhaled the traffic fumes. By the time I reached Finsbury Park it was already well past the time of my appointment. As I stood on the Victoria Line platform I could see through to the Piccadilly Line platform and it was infuriating to discover the service was now running normally, that I'd have done better to have stayed on the train at Wood Green! Doggedly I continued on my way and when I surfaced at Warren Street I managed to get a taxi. I was nearly an hour and a half late but the girls, who had received a message from Erwin, said they were very relieved to see me because they had a meeting soon. Less than fifteen minutes after my arrival at the clinic I was on my way back to the station and beginning to unwind.

I had a very touching e-mail from Ben yesterday which I printed out. It said: 'I think of you lots during this time and feel proud of you for the way that you are dealing with this illness. Writing poems days after your operation and the success in getting your poems published are tangible benchmarks of your ability to deal with what has happened. But the less obvious things – your outlook and attitude – are things that are admirable and make me feel a lot of affection and love for you. I am so lucky to have a mother with such a gift of expression of feelings and thoughts.' His words made me cry and they also made me feel very guilty because I know some of the time I have been very short-tempered with Erwin. I think I'm on a much shorter fuse immediately after the chemotherapy treatment and it would be some consolation to think the drugs are responsible or partly responsible for my behaviour. Yesterday, three days after treatment, I'm sure I was calmer than I was the previous two days. Maybe writing 'Release' has also helped.

20th May

Camellias have been in my head on and off since we had supper at the beginning of April with Henry and Helene, friends of very long standing – in fact Erwin and I each knew them separately before we met one another. On their dinner table were two pink camellia heads floating in a shallow bowl. The circles of petals in the circle of the dish were very beautiful – delicate and vulnerable somehow. They made me think of a Chinese painting, of peace. Henry insisted I took the flowers home. I kept looking at the complicated tuck of the petals in each flower-head and could find no words to describe them. Today I was looking at a UNICEF card. Its design was the Chinese word for serenity and it brought me back to the camellias again. What shade of pink is a camellia? No rose, no other flower is quite this colour. I feel there is a poem here – but what? Maybe something about taking the pink into myself – a meditation perhaps which would connect with the first part of 'The Egg of Protection' on Kate's relaxation tape. I need to develop some notes.

23rd May

Yesterday the chemotherapy session was less of an ordeal than last week. The clinic wasn't so busy, my stomach wasn't so badly upset and the whole thing was over sooner. I'm relieved that this stage is nearing its end. There are only five radiotherapy sessions left. I wish I hadn't been so anxious but I am telling myself it's not unreasonable to have been afraid of undergoing this double treatment and not to blame myself for feeling worried by it.

Myrna, whom I've known for over thirty years, has been supportive and phoned frequently during the last four months. When she was here not long ago she read the poems I've written about cancer and said she found them very moving. She asked for a copy of the sequence to keep so I printed one out. A week or so later she phoned to ask me if she could show the poems to her friend, May, who like me has been diagnosed with breast cancer. I agreed but suggested she chose the time carefully as the feelings in the poems are so strong and I was not sure how a person who had recently had surgery would react to them. Now May has written to me: 'You've been able to say what so far I haven't so that your words allow me to grieve and shout and rage over my own diagnosis and its implications.' I was moved beyond words that 'Repair' had had such an effect on someone else in the same predicament as myself. If they can help other cancer sufferers find space for their feelings then they really have achieved something worthwhile. Such a response also convinces me that I should develop the jottings in this notebook into a book.

28th May

My digestive system is badly affected by the chemotherapy. My stomach often feels churned up and eating is difficult. I rarely feel hungry but I usually feel a bit better after a small meal. However, at the moment I'm not feeling quite as exhausted by the radiotherapy as I feared I would be. It is quite clear to me now – and I wish it had been spelt out to me by a doctor – that my body will need months to recover from having part of it lopped off. I dread to think what time it will need to recuperate from these treatments. Still, I'm also aware that my body has a hoard of strength, that it harbours – I harbour – a determination to get better, to live – and as fully as possible.

There's no other reference to writing about the camellias but I have a memory of writing down visualizations which were very soothing. I must have started work on the poem very soon after my note on May 20th and it must have been finished before the end of May because I sent it with 'Release' and 'Repair' to Les Murray at the beginning of June.

The Camellias
for Helene and Henry

are floating in a shallow bowl,
circles of pink layered petals
that silence browns, saffrons, absorb
our voices, the table, the whole

room. No word for this pink
which is kinder than red, warmer
than rose, more substantial
than sunset, invites me to think

of a willow in a landscape cool
as silk, the sense of each twig,
each leaf, the pale eggshell
sky intense as the unfathomed pool

we call consciousness. I will take
the camellia colour to heart, let it
rise to my leaden head, undo
my tight jaw, smooth the ache

in my eyes. Once it's unlatched spine,
lulled stomach, encouraged knees,
put down feelers in my feet it will unfold
beyond my body, urge me to recline

on an island of pillow softness. I'll unwind
the strings of each taut kite,
watch them fly free and for a nameless
time I will float in my quiet mind.

John was in London on Wednesday and he came to see me in the evening. He has now had a second book of dementia poems published – poems in which he has edited what dementia sufferers say but added nothing of his own. People with this illness often speak in metaphor – tap directly into their inner selves. With his natural sympathy and the techniques he has worked out over the last few years John's had many meaningful communications with dementia sufferers. Often he is presented with lyrical and insightful material as individuals try to make sense of the world they now inhabit. His first book of poems *You are Words* was widely appreciated and this new book, *Openings*, is sure to reach many people too. It has a number of moving photographs of people with dementia taken by Carl Cordonnier, a well-known French photographer.

We talked about the manuscript Colin left. Maggie has sent us both copies of it and John has already read the poems. I've only glanced at them – partly because I'm still so upset about Colin's death, partly because my energy is low. John read to me several poems from *Fugue*, the sequence Colin wrote about his stay in hospital – a few of them I've seen before because he brought them to the Sunday group. As a sequence the poems provide a devastating account both of breakdown and a mental illness ward. They are so direct, alive, ironic, so aware of the predicaments of others and the obscure cleverness of some of

Colin's later work is absent. A number of poems in the manuscript are dedicated to friends and the last section of lyrical poems is dedicated to both John and me. John looked very tired and I was worried about the amount of work he is doing and the stress in his life. I wish he would protect himself more.

After my phone conversation with Grevel I sent him a copy of *Repair* and now he's written saying he thinks the sequence contains some of my best poems. He also opened up a new line of thought for me with this: 'When I came to the point in 'The Cave' where the voice reproaches you with the phrases "one-breasted" and "hardly a woman" I found myself thinking: "Ah but in ancient myths the most powerful women of all were, precisely, one-breasted." I wondered if you had looked at or might find it fruitful to look at the mythology surrounding the Amazons. They were a subject of fascination and a certain amount of fear to the ancient Greeks, at least and a very frequent image in graphic art, especially vase painting. And although very martial in their doings, they were certainly not thought of as unfeminine but rather in some odd way as too feminine for comfort. There is extensive material on them in Graves' *Greek Myths* and one recalls that Hippolyta, Theseus' queen, who turns up in *A Midsummer Night's Dream* was an Amazon. Probably other important characters in myth were one-breasted too. No doubt there are books about them. At any rate I wonder if there is something here worth looking at?'

As I read Grevel's words I had a sense of revelation – of a door opening to show a completely new vista. And the impact of the words was the stronger because they were the thoughts of an academic but approachable and sensitive man, the opposite of my judgmental father who appeared as a caricature of himself in 'The Cave'. Grevel's words have somehow changed my image of myself. It's almost like a blood transfusion. I may have lost a breast but it is true that I have gained strength. Anyone who's been through this and is continuing to live fruitfully must be stronger. This new perspective is both exciting and affirming. I can stop seeing myself as incomplete, as inferior beside all those Matisse and Picasso paintings of women. I can reduce the critical father voice that's inside my head even further.

30th May

Yesterday was a terrible day, I've caught a really nasty cold – or worse than a cold – that's affected my sinuses and throat. I felt unbelievably weak and awful. I was also worried in case I had a temperature and would have to take antibiotics which I've avoided for years. They don't agree with me at all and the last time I was on a course of antibiotic tablets they kept me awake all night. At the first chemotherapy session the pharmacist gave me antibiotics to keep at home. He explained that the treatment lowers the immune system and that I would have to take a course of pills if I caught 'flu or had a temperature. Although I've felt a bit hot and cold, I haven't, thank goodness, had a temperature, but sucking a throat lozenge and taking homeopathic Coldenza have completely upset my stomach. I was awake in the middle of the night and I lay there feeling I would never recover, never have a normal life again.

I feel less hideous today but I'm very limp and my nose and sinuses are full of infection. I have already had yesterday 'off' from the clinic because it was a bank holiday but I know I'm not fit to go up to Harley Street today. When I phoned the clinic the radiotherapist I spoke to was concerned that I was missing today even though I explained I wouldn't have dreamt of cancelling without good reason. Apart from anything else I really want treatment finished. There are only two sessions left.

31st May

The cold has moved down to my throat now and I have a bit of a cough but I can see I must go to the clinic today. I'm due to have the mid-way blood test and the chemotherapy nurses want to check my health. I don't have a temperature and I shall absolutely resist it if they try to give me antibiotics. I feel extremely fed up and unwell. Luckily the weather is warmer so I shouldn't get chilled going out. I still feel frightened, as if recovery is completely beyond my reach; it's been hard to keep going with bits of work during the last few days but I know it would be much worse if I hadn't. I've drafted a letter to send out to people who might be interested in the Writing for Self-Discovery course John and I are doing in November. I've also managed to do some notes for 'Seaweed', the next section in the narrative poem. It's a vision. Katie, the main character, dreams she is on different beaches she knows including the beach she lived near to as a child. The beaches melt into one another. I suspect I have too much material, especially about the beach from her childhood. Still, writing notes about sea and beach, especially using the beach I played on as a child and being taken out in a rowing boat by my father, has been therapeutic. That memory of my father is a good one. He was relaxed, jolly and as the rowing boat went up over the crests of high waves I remember having a wonderful feeling of adventure. I've been reading quite a bit and have finished Kate Atkinson's *Behind the Scenes at the Museum*. I like the way she deals with time, memory, different perspectives. At one point she calls memory 'a lost property office'. Mimi told me American poet Lucille Clifton has written poems about breast cancer. I've looked up her book and there is one about losing a breast which is very lyrical and moving.

1st June

They were good at the clinic yesterday, got a doctor to check me over and although one of the young nurses brought up the dread word *antibiotics*, the doctor was definitive: it wouldn't serve any purpose. I had the last radiotherapy treatment today. I'm glad it's over and would feel more upbeat about this if I wasn't so weary.

CHAPTER TEN

The After Effects
of Double Treatment

3rd June 2000

The treatments have left me feeling utterly exhausted, demoralized and very low. This morning I spent quite a while crying. I know what I've been through is for my own protection but I feel as if my body's been badly abused. It's helped me a little to let some of this out to Ruth and Mimi over the phone. I also spoke to a counsellor on the Breast Cancer Care Helpline who said: 'That saying about all the stuffing being knocked out of you takes on a completely new meaning, doesn't it?' She confirmed that it could take weeks to get over, longer for the exhaustion from radiotherapy to wear off. This fact wasn't mentioned in the 'After Effects' section of the leaflet about radiotherapy I was given at the clinic. I've been very well treated there but I shall send in a comment on this omission.

5th June

I saw Kate on Saturday after a gap of weeks – with the daily journey up to the clinic it would have been too much to fit in other daytime appointments. At the moment I feel it's my body that needs help most and that as far as counselling is concerned, it's best to draw on the skills I've gained from her over the years. She gave me a massage which was very gentle but I was aware that every part of me felt so frail and so tensed up it could hardly even bear her calming hands. I unwound a little. Today I had a second massage and was able to relax much more. I really felt the benefit afterwards. My sore throat is slowly improving and food is tasting marginally better. I've managed to do more work on the narrative poem and I've been thinking about Grevel's letter – his comments about the Amazons.

12th June

I am sitting on a bed at the clinic. I should be starting the next cycle of chemotherapy but I still feel extremely weak and as my stomach has continued to be disturbed I feel generally awful. In my opinion I'm not fit to undergo treatment today. I've explained this to the sister who listened sympathetically and said she agreed with me even though my blood count was all right. She's gone off to confirm with the oncologist that treatment should be postponed for a week. I still keep feeling overcome by a hopeless fear that I'll never be strong again but I'm fighting it. Somehow I managed to run and enjoy two classes last week though I found them tiring, especially the second one. I think I need to hoard my grains of energy more carefully.

13th June

I didn't have any treatment yesterday. The sister said I was exhausted from the mix of radiotherapy and chemotherapy and eating less than half the amount I normally do. She gave me boxes of fruit flavoured drinks packed with proteins, minerals etc., as a food supplement. I can see now that I should have phoned in for advice sooner but it simply hadn't occurred to me that there was anything they could do. I am going to be quite strict with myself about resting, do everything I can to build myself up for chemotherapy next Monday.

16th June

The proofs of the *Parents* anthology have arrived and Dilys is sending contributors copies of their poems and their biographical notes. A couple of days ago the poems for the competition organized by the Writers Conference at Winchester turned up. Although I had to cancel running workshops and giving a talk at this conference, which takes place in a couple of weeks, I agreed I would still judge the competition. There were more poems than I expected and the deadline I've been given is only just over a week away so I'm getting on with it as quickly as I can. I've already spent several hours on it and so far only found a few good or goodish poems. Luckily I'm a little stronger – it's such a relief not to feel completely under everything, to have my stomach calmer. I still have a tickly cough so I've been putting a bowl of hot water with a drop or two of tea tree oil in it in my room – a friend's suggestion. This definitely has a soothing effect.

Yesterday I talked to Mary MacRae on the phone. I first met her last autumn when she came to interview me for *Magma* magazine. She was very complimentary about my work and I discovered that she'd attended Mimi's versification course and other Poetry School courses. I agreed to give her a tutorial early in the new year and when she sent in work at Christmas time I thought it had much potential. I also realized from two of the poems that she'd had cancer. Because of my illness the tutorial didn't take place until March. After it we had a long chat partly about cancer but other things too. Since March Mary and I have talked on the phone sometimes. She's sympathetic and I find it extremely comforting to share thoughts with someone I know who went through a similar experience a year or so before me. When she was ill she didn't know anyone who'd recently had breast cancer whom she could turn to. Yesterday we talked about everyone going through times when they feel they are unable to cope. I found this very reassuring and appreciate the time she's so willingly given me.

There is no other reference in my notebook to the Amazons or developing a poem but Grevel's letter, my new perspective and drafting 'Amazon' helped to sustain me during this difficult time. I know it was written by the middle of June. Here's the final version:

Amazon
for Grevel

For four months
all those Matisse and Picasso women
draped against
plants, balconies, Mediterranean Sea, skies
have taunted me
with the beautiful globes of their breasts as I've filled

my emptiness
with pages of scrawl, with fecund May, its floods
of green, its irrepressible
wedding-lace white, buttercup gold,
but failed to cover
the image of myself as a misshapen clown

until you reminded me
that in Greek myth the most revered women
were the single-breasted
Amazons who mastered javelins, bows, rode
horses into battle,
whose fierce queens were renowned for their femininity.

Then recognizing the fields I'd fought my way across
I raised my shield
of glistening words, saw it echoed the sun.

20th June

Yesterday was a boiling hot day but somehow I got through the ordeal of chemotherapy. My stomach was so badly affected I found it almost impossible to eat and food is still unpalatable today. Ben had the bright idea that we could hire an air conditioning machine which Erwin did with some difficulty. However, we couldn't make it work. While it was whirring away it was actually making the room warmer which was funny in a grotesque way. Today's my birthday and I was touched by all the kind cards and presents I received. The day hasn't seemed very birthday-like because I've felt so ghastly.

22nd June

I phoned up the clinic yesterday because I'm still finding it very difficult to eat and they urged me to take some additional anti-sickness pills which they gave me not long ago. I took one dose but I still felt very queasy during the night. Someone has been to look at the air conditioning machine. The reason it wasn't working was because the suction tube wasn't actually attached! Now we've sorted this out the weather, needless to say, isn't particularly hot. We've had to hire the machine for a month but I bet there won't be any more very hot days while it's here!

Yesterday evening Angie came over after work for a short time. She is always quietly sympathetic and calming and it was lovely to see her. Her manner and her conscientiousness make her a gifted speech therapist. She brought me the perfect birthday present: a lavender sleep mask – a sachet inside a bag which is deep purple velvet on one side and white cotton patterned with lavender flowers on the other. The mask can be placed over the forehead and eyes for ten minutes or so while you are lying down. I've already tried it and it's wonderful, soft and soothing and makes me visualize lavender bushes in flower. It's comforting too just to hold the bag in my hands and stroke it as if it's a silken-backed animal.

27th June

Yesterday I got through the second session of cycle four of the chemo-therapy. Even before she saw the blood test results the sister said I looked pale and that she thought my red blood corpuscles were down. She was right and I wasn't very surprised to hear that I'm anaemic. The count was just above the point at which they normally give a blood transfusion but she felt that a blood transfusion would be a good idea. I have been holding down a dreadful fear that I simply wouldn't have the strength to cope with two more cycles of treatment. The oncologist confirmed the blood transfusion and it was an enormous relief to be told it would give me a boost that would carry me through the last two stages of the treatment. So for some hours tomorrow blood will be fed into me drop by drop. I'm not looking forward to it one bit even though I'm glad I'm getting this help. Apparently I should begin to feel a difference in a few days. I found it difficult to sleep but I held Angie's lavender bag to my face, breathed in the smell of lavender, imagined bees murmuring in lavender bushes.

2nd July

The last few days have been very hard. I found the blood transfusion taxing. It made me queasy – I think the process was a shock to my body. Anyway it was a strain to spend hours on both Monday and Wednesday at the clinic attached to a drip. By Wednesday evening I was so exhausted I felt I couldn't cope with anything. Perhaps because I was over-tired I slept badly and my stomach was upset. I'm keen to cut off from the treatments as much as I possibly can and focus on the narrative poem, books and other ideas. All the way through this ordeal, and even now at this very low point, writing has separated me from it. As I sit down to work on a poem I have a sense of pushing down the illness, refusing it room, stepping out of it. While I am writing – whether I manage ten minutes or an hour – I am not an ill person, I am my whole self; and this is so whether what I am writing is connected with cancer or not. Writing has been my protection and salvation. Back in May I wrote a piece for the Second Light Newsletter about how I've used writing to support myself. I found it very validating to do this.

3rd July

Scintilla arrived last Thursday and it gave me a lift to see the whole of the *Repair* sequence including 'The Cave' in it. The journal also has 'Knitting', a royal sonnet sequence by Mary, which won third prize in the *Scintilla* poetry competition. It's moving and accomplished, looks at the patterns or non-patterns of life through connections between herself, her mother and daughter and brings in her experience of cancer. I had a long chat with Anne Cluysenaar on the phone yesterday evening. It is very encouraging to know a poet and critic of her calibre is excited by my work.

4th July

The blood transfusion must be taking effect as I'm beginning to feel I have a little more energy. I'm still determined to extract every ounce I can out of life and the end of the treatment doesn't feel so far out of reach now. Often in the past few weeks I've felt I was just hanging on, that I've been saved by the minutes of concentration I've managed to muster to write the narrative poem and read the proofs of *Parents* or carried by the sympathy of the person I'm talking to. If I think about it those minutes of being immersed in something positive also include the books I've been reading, listening to tapes of tranquil music and picking fruit in the garden. The raspberries, in particular, have been lusciously pink and abundant this year and there is something life-giving about picking them, finding I can enjoy eating a few mouthfuls at supper time or putting a boxful away in the freezer for the winter. All these things have helped me to keep sane, to hold onto living, its gold dust. Visualizations, which I've done almost every day, have also been helpful in calming me down and have led to writing ideas. The main new one is round lavender and was set off by the lavender sleep mask which Angie brought.

Lavender: Note

Beds of it, Provence fields and the market in Arles with lavender bags, great bowls of loose lavender, lavender soaps, bees humming in summer herbaceous borders among the hollyhocks, marguerites, phlox, delphiniums and sucking nectar. I'll get Erwin to see what he can find on the Internet about lavender – its history and healing powers. I think there is a poem to write though quite what hasn't yet emerged. Kindness should be part of it.

6th July

Dilys spent several hours here on Tuesday so that we could start choosing poems to put forward to Gladys Mary Coles for the anthology of women's poetry. To save my energy I sat propped up on my bed and we discussed and picked out a number of poems. I had a short rest before lunch and again in the afternoon. During this time Dilys went on with the shortlisting of poems. She is so generous – arrived with flowers and cakes. We have set aside more dates to go on with the selection process.

I was suddenly aware of what felt like an ulcer in my mouth yesterday. It was very painful by the time of the Prose and Poetry workshop in the evening but a paracetamol and the lively work people brought helped me through the session. In the middle of the night I woke up to find my tongue was swollen and the pain now extended into my ear which was worrying. I was also angry – it seemed as if yet another problem had come along to slap me down. However, a second painkiller, doing visualizations and thinking about section nineteen of the narrative poem, carried me through the night. I suppose I must have drifted in and out of sleep. Today I can hardly bear food in my mouth at all which seems very hard now that I'm beginning to feel like eating.

I went to the clinic as early as I could – I was due to go there today anyway for the 'low point' blood test. My blood count is satisfactory again which is good but it was difficult to focus on this when I felt so uncomfortable. A doctor prescribed two different mouthwashes followed by a thick yellowy concoction – also to be swilled round the mouth. Apparently I have a mouth infection rather than an ulcer. I waited ages for the medicines because they were short-staffed and I felt increasingly tense but somehow managed to revise quite a lot of section eighteen of the narrative poem. The journey home added to the strain. The tube was very full so I sat on the floor which prompted someone to give up their seat. I've followed the instructions about using the mouthwashes very carefully and this evening I detected a small improvement but eating is still extremely painful and I still feel 'struck down'.

The weather is very oppressive. However, the courgettes and tomatoes in the garden like it and are growing like mad. The raspberries are amazing. It's only twenty-four hours since I picked them but more have ripened. Seeds from the goosegrass growing among the canes attach themselves to my trousers whenever I pick fruit. The way they cling to the material when I try to brush them off makes me think of myself clinging on.

9th July

My mouth cleared up over Friday and Saturday. I suppose I wouldn't have been so het up if I'd known that the problem could be resolved quite quickly. All in all though I feel utterly wearied and I've lost a lot of confidence.

Dumping

I'm fed up with having my body poisoned.
I'm fed up with having to cancel things.
I'm fed up with feeling weak.
I'm fed up with having a disturbed stomach.
I'm fed up with the attacks on my mouth and the skin of my hands.
I'm fed up with unexpected new problems.
I'm fed up that eating's still quite a misery.
I'm fed up that there are still two more cycles.
I'm fed up that I can do so little.
I'm fed up with being cut off.
I'm fed up with being dependent on help.
I'm fed up with being a drag on Erwin.

CHAPTER ELEVEN

The Final Cycles of Chemotherapy

17th July 2000

I am writing with my left hand as my right arm is soaking in hot water, a preliminary to chemotherapy as it brings up the veins and makes it easier to insert the cannula for the drugs. During the last week or so I have felt considerably stronger and on Wednesday, by having a rest every now and then, I managed to put in quite a long day with Dilys selecting poems to put forward for the women's anthology. On Thursday I had a massage with Kate which I found very restful and on Friday I gave a tutorial.

18th July

The chemotherapy session yesterday went smoothly and I don't feel so knocked down by it as I did by the June treatments. Once I'd had the initial blood test instead of staying at the clinic for the drugs to be prepared I went out with Erwin. On the corner of Marylebone High Street we found what called itself the Love Café. It's in Aveda, a shop selling body lotions and flowers, and it has excellent coffee and wholefoods. It was a sunny morning and sitting in the café eating toast made from substantial brown bread with splendid jams and looking at the striped awning across the street, I suddenly had a sense of being on holiday. It was wonderful pretending I was free – on a day out. This small diversion put me in a completely different frame of mind.

Lavender: Note

I'm thinking about a poem in three parts:

(a)   A visualization round the lavender sleep bag Angie brought me – its colour, scent, texture, what it makes me think of – bees in bushes etc.

(b)   The pale mauve of the long lavender fields in Provence, the lavender bags and soaps in Arles market, maybe bringing in van Gogh and also the old woman I saw in Arles market whom I've written about in a poem I've abandoned.

(c)   The way the purple lavender bag reminds me of the work with words Angie and I have done at Flightways. Lavender has a clarity that goes with Angie's dedication. A major theme in my next collection of poetry will be communication as this is one of the subjects of the narrative poem. The lavender poem will connect with this.

Most of my writing energy was going into the narrative poem at this point and it was nine months before I developed these notes. When I did I found myself describing chemotherapy directly. Perhaps at some level I knew I couldn't tackle the subject head on until the treatment was far behind me. After much experimentation and some feedback from John I produced three separate poems because the subject matter didn't connect well enough to make one poem. My thoughts about Angie fitted best into the first poem. The second poem began in a Provence lavender field and then shifted to the market in Arles and the old woman. The third idea became a poem about words and teaching people who had almost no speech. Here is the first poem:

Lavender
for Angie

With a sachet of lavender secreted inside it
the purple bag is plump as a small bird's
breast, echoes your voice, its restful
clarity. When I slide my thumb down
the velvet underside a sense of psalm

fills me and dark cat night sidling in,
fitting the mound of herself to
a human back. I picture tension easing
in the day-to-day shifts we make
with those we're knitted to. Though I'm weak

the emperor purple gloves my skin
awake, rallies the brain's metropolis, sends
pungent messages to the pulsing townships.
For months my braced body's fought
the indiscriminate battalions sent in to rout

any cancerous cell filching a plot
of land but now it's flagging, wants
to hunch in a ditch, weep at its wounds.
Useless to wish frailty was a boiler suit
I could unbutton – it's married to the roots

of my hair, my blood. But this pouch
you chose for me, its insistent coolth,
raises a garden where flowering bushes
are blue-leaved and threaded with bee thrum,
raspberries spill ripeness on my thumbs.

21st July

This week has continued to go more easily in spite of the treatment though yesterday I woke feeling exhausted and low. Nevertheless I managed to do quite a bit of work on the narrative poem. I'm trying to work out where to stop the story and end the poem and last week I drafted section nineteen, 'Scissors'. The main climax of the poem is in this part. It's brought about by William, a bright lad, who has a severe speech impediment and can't walk as a result of cerebral palsy. He's difficult partly because he's over-protected by his harassed mum and in the 'Scissors' section he expresses his anger by crawling upstairs to her bedroom and cutting up some garments she's made. He then smears them with cream from her dressing table. Most of the sections are written in the voice of one of the four main characters. William's sections are what he writes or dreams about and 'Scissors' is his gleeful account on the computer of the havoc he's created in his mother's bedroom. I sifted through dozens of dramatic – mainly over-dramatic – ideas for the form his rebellion would take but nothing felt right until I hit on the cutting up of the clothes. I'm now planning section twenty and there will only be one more. I'm thinking about a title for the whole poem. Something about the voice in the box maybe because by the end William has a communicator – a sophisticated computer which speaks what he keys into it. This kind of title would fit too because most of the characters communicate more directly by the end of the poem.

Although this illness and the treatments have been such an ordeal I feel more than ever that life is good and this has helped me to hang on and squeeze what I can out of everything. I'm beginning to feel excited about reaching the end of the treatment – can see I am going to escape from the trap I'm in. With luck the chemo will be over by this time next month and all I'll need is patience while I regain strength. I'm longing to go away which we will, I hope, do early in September. We already have the brochures of some possible hotels in the Cotswolds and Eastbourne. Of course we won't book anything until I feel confident I'm well enough to enjoy being away from home. It was very hard to accept that I'm not strong enough to make the relatively short journey in three weeks to do a reading for Poetry Suffolk but I'm looking forward to the launch of *Parents* on September 21st and my new and selected poems in October. Besides, Poetry Suffolk is going to re-book me for next year and two other events I've had to cancel have led to fixtures for next summer. I've also written a proposal to do a workshop and reading in Dorchester round *Parents*. I realize I must be careful though not to overdo things during the autumn and winter.

26th July

I've now completed cycle five of the treatment and I still have a feeling of uplift even though the session this Monday rather flattened me. However, I had a sleep for two hours yesterday afternoon and felt much better afterwards. I think I'm continuing to gain strength as I get further away from the radiotherapy. Of course I must be getting the benefit of the blood transfusion too. It was great to feel well enough to go to the theatre on Saturday afternoon.

3rd August

I've now finished 'Voice', section twenty of the narrative poem, and am planning the final part so I'm coming to the end of more than a year's work – much more if I include the sporadic notemaking I did for a couple of years before I began detailed planning. I need to bring the Anglo-Saxon church at Deerhurst into the last section and I've been visualizing the visit we made to it about fifteen years ago: looking across an August cornfield, the smell of sun and grain, the old farm and barn nearby, the church as if untouched for centuries and remote, though in fact it was only a few miles from Tewkesbury. I remember too the cool and light inside the building and its Saxon features: an apse, two narrow, arched windows and a carved angel, also the flood of heat as we came out of the church, a sense of being rooted in the past, of perfect quiet.

On Sunday morning Erwin tripped over a paving stone as we set off for a walk and fell very heavily on his arm. He was quite shocked and his elbow was still so painful after lunch he went by taxi to Casualty in Barnet General Hospital. It was a hot close day. At half past eight Erwin called to say he'd had to wait for three hours in the crowded and stifling waiting room before his arm was X-rayed and that it took three attempts. The young doctor who saw him was exhausted. He was told nothing was broken. He arrived home with his arm in an elasticated bandage and a sling. On Monday he couldn't even hold his glasses because his wrist hurt so much. This morning huge bruises have appeared. However, his wrist is improving every day and he can move his arm more. I'm glad I'm stronger because I've obviously had to do more and we are hampered by his not being able to drive.

I had a lovely letter from Les Murray yesterday in reply to the one I'd sent him in June in which I'd said I felt awkward blurting out my news about my illness at Mimi's launch. I'd also explained how much writing had been supporting me and enclosed some of the cancer poems. In his letter he said that my news had shocked him but that it was infinitely worse for me for whom it wasn't merely news. He's taken six poems for *Quadrant*: 'Today There Is Time', 'Bath', 'The Shell', 'Release', 'The Camellias' and 'The Cave'. Best of all he remarked: 'You've written very bravely and with no less skill under what must have been awful conditions.' This comment from such an outstanding poet lifted my heart to the sky. In connection with my new book, *Insisting on Yellow*, he wrote: 'I love that colour. Porsche yellow's what I call my favourite shade: what's yours?' I don't know how to answer that question because I love so many yellows. The more I think about it the more different yellows crowd into my head.

4th August

We were surprised and a bit worried that Erwin was called back to the hospital. It turns out that there is a hairline fracture in his arm. Luckily it doesn't need to be put in plaster or have any other treatment but he must keep the sling on some of the time. When I had the nadir blood test yesterday the count was low for the first time. I gathered from the nurse who gave me the result that it was not especially low but of course it made me feel a bit anxious that the white cells won't recover sufficiently before the next treatment though she assured me this was unlikely to be a problem. I shall do plenty of visualizations of white cells dancing around, kicking up their legs and generally asserting themselves. It would be such a downer if I can't finish off the chemotherapy by August 21st!

8th August

Dilys and I put in a good day of work yesterday. We did some publicity planning for the *Parents* anthology. Some readings are already fixed and there are others in the pipeline. The complicated proofs are finally finished. The book has meant a great deal of work for Stephen at Enitharmon Press especially as there are one hundred and fourteen contributors and many details to check up on. There is something of a question mark about the book being ready in time for the launch but we must keep our nerve and hope all will be well!

Heather, a friend from school and her husband Gerald came for the day from Oxford on Sunday. We don't meet very often now and it was lovely to catch up.

Seeing Heather made me think of Chichester where my family moved when I was fourteen. I found myself thinking of the South Downs where I often went for walks with my sister, parents or friends – how we had to go to the far end of our lane and tramp for a mile and a half past cornfields and farms on narrow hedgerowed roads where hips, haws and spindleberries were abundant in the autumn. Sometimes we took a picnic with us and went down into the next narrow valley and climbed Bow Hill which has a thick covering of yew bushes on its side. The last part of this ascent is a scramble up steep chalky paths and over turf where tormentil, scabious and harebells grow. This is the landscape of my teens. My feelings were in such a tangle at that time. Sometimes I was intensely excited by everything but often I was hopelessly cast down or knotted up with anxiety. Walking on the Downs was always a release. I miss fields, hedges, hills and the sea even though we have the park behind our house. This is another reason why I am longing to go away.

17th August

My blood count was all right on Monday but the treatment upset my stomach a lot and really pulled me down. I know there's not much further to go but I am absolutely fed up with chemotherapy and its invasion of my life. I am well into the last section of the narrative poem. I'm still gauging the exact point where I'm going to stop. This last part presents more problems with structure than any other section. I am definitely going to call the poem 'Voicebox'.

Poem note

The words and images haven't come to me yet but I want to write about a car that's been abandoned in the park. Every day I walk past it and every day it's been more vandalised: the tyres let down, the windows shattered, the upholstery torn out, everything inside it tampered with. It was a shock today to see it burnt out. I imagine teenagers must have set it on fire last night. The air still smelt acrid with smoke and it's reduced to a rusting skeleton. This kind of destruction is so mindless, vicious – the opposite of holding onto life, being creative, of everything I believe in.

21st August: Wow!

My last chemotherapy session took place today and it went easily. The nurse who injected the drugs was sweet – raised her arm and said 'Hooray' when she'd finished. Part of me hasn't taken in yet that it actually is over. For the last six months I've braced myself day after day to face this treatment and to hold a sense of dread at bay. I suppose it will take a while for me to unwind. In our 'break' before the chemo we went to the Love Café and then round the corner to Daunt's in Marylebone High Street. This is a beautiful bookshop. I bought *An Anthropologist on Mars* by Oliver Sacks. I like his way of writing. It's alive and alert and his scientific investigations are written in accessible language. The first account in this book is of an artist who went colour blind. The effect this had on him, how he adapts to the situation and uses it to develop his painting is fascinating. I am wondering again about writing some poems which focus on colour. The first might be about the blind girl I saw in the Chagall Museum in Nice.

On Saturday I did a reading to illustrate the possibilities of narrative poetry. This followed on from a Second Light workshop at the Torriano Meeting House in Kentish Town. Everyone was very receptive. I was conscious too how much stronger I am than I was when I did the competition adjudication there at the end of February. The appreciative comments afterwards were uplifting and the afternoon made me feel normal life is just round the corner. I'm putting a bit of pressure on myself to finish drafting 'Voicebox' and send it to Caroline by this Saturday.

Poem note

To celebrate the end of treatment – an extravaganza? – this went through my head:

When it's all over I'm going to open all my windows and shout hallelujah,
when it's all over I'll stand on the roof and sing *Land of Hope and Glory*,
when it's all over I'll loudspeaker my news from a van down these roads of plastic Greek urns and tubs of geraniums,
when it's over I'll ring everyone up in the middle of the night,
when it's all over I'll make sixteen bowls of summer pudding,
leap like a kangaroo, spout like a whale, wallow like a hippopotamus,
fill the sky with fireworks,
when it's all over I'll do none of these things –
I'll climb back to strength word by word.

CHAPTER TWELVE

Escape to Eastbourne and Book Launches

25th August 2000

If I can make a poem from my answer to Les' question about my favourite yellow it would fit into a series about colour. Yellows I find crucial are: my yellow teapot, the comfortable yellows of our kitchen cupboards, the moon, butter dripping, van Gogh's yellows, the yellow headscarf a brain damaged client of mine wore, the yellow badge the Nazis forced Jews to wear. I need to go further with this.

28th August

I've celebrated the end of my treatment by developing 'When It's All Over'. I didn't feel up to any other kind of celebration – maybe this is more special. I was really pleased to use 'Pacific Palisades' because I love the alliteration of the name and the images it conjures up. I've only heard of this town, which is an outlying part of Los Angeles on the coast between Santa Monica and Malibu, because it's the home of Lance Lee, a poet I became friendly with a couple of years ago after we did a reading together. I like the emotional pitch of his writing, the way he explores feelings and uses natural imagery.

When It's All Over

I'm going to throw open my windows and yell: 'hallelujah',
dial up friends in the middle of the night to give them
the glad tidings, e-mail New South Wales and Pacific Palisades,
glorify the kitchen by making sixteen summer puddings,
watch blackberry purple soak slowly into
the bread and triumph over the curved glass of the bowls.

When it's all over I'll feed my cracked skin
with lavender and aloe vera, lower my exhausted body into
foaming cream, a sweetness of honey and let it wallow,
reward it with a medal, beautify it with garlands of thornless roses,
wrap it in sleep. Then from tents of blurred dreams
I'll leap like a kangaroo, spout like a whale.

Once it's over I'm going to command my computer to bellow
Land of Hope and Glory, loudspeaker my news
down these miles of orderly streets where the houses wear
mock Tudor beams and plastic Greek columns, dance
the Highland Fling in front of controlled tubs of cockerel geraniums,
sigh with enormous satisfaction when I make the evening headlines.

When it's finally over I'm going to gather these fantasies,
fling them into my dented and long lost college trunk,
dump it in the unused cellar
        climb back to strength
        up my rope of words.

Reading this now I think it carries the energy I was longing to regain. Writing it made me feel powerful, extravagant. I sent it to Steven Blyth, the editor of *Prop*, who'd contacted me out of the blue asking if I would submit poems for the magazine. He immediately accepted it. Ruth gave a copy of it to a close friend of hers who was seriously ill. Her friend was so taken with the poem and encouraged by it she showed it to everybody who came to see her. I was overwhelmed that my words offered such support to a sick person. That 'rope of words' did help me climb back to health but the journey turned out to be slow and difficult.

My stomach and bowels are still in turmoil from the treatment last week. It must be the accumulative effect of the chemo. Although I've managed to separate my creativity from illness and made something out of the experience, my body has often found it very difficult to bear. The whole marathon – from the day I was called back to the hospital at the beginning of January – has been a stark reminder of how short life is, how easily it can be lost. The corollary to that, of course, is not to waste a moment of it. Time is gold dust.

We've now booked to go to Eastbourne on 12th September for five days. This gives me as much time as possible to build up my strength before we go and also to recover after we get back and organize myself for the first writing workshop of the academic year on September 20th and the launch of *Parents* on the following day. We're now expecting the book five or six days in advance of the launch. U.A. Fanthorpe, who has written the preface, has agreed to introduce it. I'm going to give a brief overview of the book – its different sections and how I linked the poems. Then ten contributors will read their poems.

3rd September

I've continued to feel worse than I did in the weeks before the final chemo session – tired all the time and sometimes I can't shake off the fear that I'll never regain my energy.

7th September

Note for the colour poems

Water has no shape of its own, no colour of its own but it has the ability to take on other colours brilliantly or subtly. It often distorts, sometimes enhances what it reflects. The light and colour changes in water echo changing moods.

My stomach is still disturbed and even though I knew my return to strength would be slow I find it hard to accept. I'm longing to get on with my life. Why am I moaning? Here I am writing this on the tube on my way to meet Caroline. When I saw her in June I was in bed and after fifty minutes hardly up to speaking! We're going to have a snack and I'm giving her the final sections of 'Voicebox' and she'll comment on the whole piece. I've started developing notes for a poem about the blind girl in the Chagall Museum but I'm finding it difficult to decide how to approach it.

13th September

I'm writing on the tube again. We're on our way to Eastbourne. We *really* are on our way! Yesterday was horrible. First of all there was the fuel crisis which meant hardly any petrol was being delivered to garages. Erwin set off early on a petrol hunt and I went to see the doctor about my digestive system. If I don't take Milpar I'm constipated, if I do I have near-diarrhoea all day. The doctor was running very late and my stomach felt particularly rebellious during the wait but I was relieved when he said the problem was almost certainly due to the chemotherapy and not something else. He prescribed Fybogel and a syrup that's even milder than Milpar.

15th September

Yesterday we walked to Beachy Head. The first mile or so was along the esplanade and I was amused by the large gulls walking on the shingle with a distinctive gait. A miniature train chugged past us. 'It's for the kiddies,' said Erwin but it was full of white-haired oldies on their way to the café at the terminus. A path took us upwards through rocky gardens, then we continued climbing on a road that passed a turreted Victorian mansion which emitted the sounds and even the smell of school. The foot of the Downs brought us to a full stop. Ahead a steep chalky path beckoned me to scramble up it, to forget that I still find the stairs at home tiring. I noticed the road veered off to the left but I was determined not to take it and I started to climb. Of course I was soon breathless but it didn't matter because the view behind us was opening out. We kept turning round and taking rests on the short turf until at last we could see the bandstand, the seafront hotels, the pier on its thin legs, the town stretching inland and miles of sea that changed from postcard blue to indigo, green and grey as the wind blew clouds in front of the sun. I made out a tiny boat, then the sun silvered everything. We climbed higher through scrubland with haw-thorns, elderberries trailing traveller's joy and brambles and at last emerged on the open Downs. I relished taking lungfuls of fresh air and with every step I felt I was defying illness, trampling it underfoot.

Suddenly we could see the sea to our right as well as our left and far ahead were seven cliffs which I knew must be the Seven Sisters. The first looked like a compressed Camembert cheese with white innards oozing out. Soon we were walking towards one of the crumbling faces of Beachy Head – its hanging walls and chimneys shone dramatically in the sun. I'd walked at least five miles.

20th September

Soon after we arrived home on Monday Dilys phoned to tell me copies of *Parents* hadn't yet arrived. The launch is three days away. I've just had an e-mail from Stephen and the books have arrived. This is my first big public occasion since I've been ill. I know I'll enjoy the evening but I need to limit the time I attend because I'm still weak.

I feel plunged back into life. Caroline has sent comments on 'Voicebox' and she's very positive about it. She's made suggestions for revision but none of them are drastic.

24th September

The launch was a success. The events room at the top of Waterstone's in Piccadilly holds one hundred and fifty people and it was almost full. The book looks absolutely splendid with David Hockney's painting, *My Parents*, on the cover set against an indigo background. U.A. Fanthorpe spoke warmly about the anthology and the poems. Some of those read were very emotional and seemed to make a considerable impact on the audience. Lots of people came to talk to me afterwards, enthusiastic about the book and pleased to see me out and about again. I stayed longer than I intended and went home tired but satisfied.

My digestive system is settling down better but my hair still looks pale and wispy. I can't think what I can do with it before the launch of *Insisting on Yellow*. I suppose it will be ages before it thickens and begins to feel and look like hair again. I'm also worried – and I've felt worried on and off for months – that I've done nothing about my two teeth which broke a couple of weeks after the operation. I still don't feel fit enough to face having much work done at the dentist.

I wrote back to Les at the beginning of the month and asked him what shade of yellow Porsche yellow was. I also told him how writing had supported me and enabled me to step outside my ill body. As I'd just finished the celebration poem I put it in with the letter. I've now had a card back from him – he has a knack of squeezing addresses into a tiny rectangle and including more matter on the rest of the card than most people do in a two-page letter. He said he liked my letter and poem and that he planned to print the latter. In answer to my question he wrote: '*Porsche yellow* may be a bit imaginary. There are two classic German yellows, the buttercup of Hohenzollern and the rich egg-yolk yellow of Habsburg, and I favour the latter. Porsche paints cars in both and I love an intermediate shade they use, between the two, so it's a personal thing of mine. Good luck if you versify it.' When I read this splendid explanation I knew without a doubt that I must write the yellow poem.

26th September

The walk to Beachy Head has stayed in my head. I wrote about it in detail partly to hang onto it because I had a feeling it would lead to a poem. It could connect with the colour idea – the different colours we saw, especially the changing colours of the sea and also with recovery, being alive.

2nd October

I'm not finding this recovery and readjustment period easy. It's true that I do have noticeably more strength now but it depresses me that it will be some while before I return to something like normal. After all I've already been sidelined for over eight months. I reached a sort of crisis point at the weekend partly, I think, because I was tired after doing rather a lot. I'd held the first three-hour sessions of my new workshop, 'The Writing Process', which is one thing I feel buoyant about – I think it's going to work very well indeed. Everyone is committed and enthusiastic and the standard of writing is high. However, because the session was demanding I found myself worrying that I might not be up to running the 'Writing for Self-Discovery' weekend course with John next month and then slept badly. I've had a talk with Ruth who encouraged me to be patient and careful for a while longer. I can see I must concentrate on what I most want to do i.e. work and readings and let other things go. In a consultation session with Kate last week we looked at the fact that I tended to focus on what I'd not done and to brush aside what I have done. I can see that emotionally I get fixated on deprivation – what's not been given to me, what's wrong, what I've lost, what I've always been without. I can also see I often discount – though not as much as I used to – achievements, everything that is satisfying. It's as if my normal state is to be deprived. I know this attitude is left from the past and that I need to work to change this mindset because it's controlling me. Nevertheless it is trying, upsetting even that I can't just roll on with ordinary life.

6th October

Notes for poem about yellow

Because I've insisted on yellow you write to me about your favourite shade, that mix of the buttercup of Hohenzollern and the rich egg-yolk of Habsburg, ask what shade I prefer. And the yellows come crowding in: primrose fragile as warmth in February; buttercups in the fields opposite my childhood house above the Clyde, those petals we shone on our chins or sold as food in the shop we set up on a green bench; my yellow kitchen cupboards, the colour fraying at the edges; the chrome stripes on curtains I once seamed on my mother-in-law's sewing machine; the Mediterranean yellow of the lemons in the dish I brought home from Taormina; the neatly-pitted skin of real lemon and its satisfying zest, tartness; that yellow badge I was lucky enough to know nothing about as I watched warships sailing down the Firth to war. The fierce yellow of sunflower petals radiating from tight circles of seeds, the flowers heaving themselves as if to compete with the sun; the sun turning tree trunks, grass, tarmac paths to gold in September. Wouldn't our time be better spent if we put down all our weapons and meditated on yellow?

13th October

Insisting on Yellow reached Stephen yesterday and he posted me a copy which arrived this morning. I am THRILLED with it. The book is a joy to look at. On the front cover is a painting by Adrian Berg, *Cambridge Gate, Regent's Park, late November 1988*. This is very gold, almost abstract with a suggestion of pink flowers and orange-red suns and it reflects the impression of the phoenix in the title poem so exactly it could be a response to reading the poem. The painting is set against a rich green and black and the two colours are repeated on the back. The printer was later than expected in delivering it and I've felt worried all week that it wouldn't arrive in time for the launch on Sunday. Now everything's in place!

This image came into my head: 'all the gold embroidery of pain'. I know I have more cancer poems to write but meanwhile I am well on in the revision of 'Voicebox'. I've just heard that the closing date for the *Scintilla* poetry competition has been extended from October 1st to November 1st. This is one of the very few competitions that doesn't have a length limit and it's too good an opportunity to miss so I've made up my mind to enter it. It's something of a pressure to finish off the poem but it's worth it.

21st October

The thirty-six hours before the launch were rather depressing because at least twelve people phoned, all very apologetic that illness or another problem meant they couldn't come. By Saturday afternoon I was in a panic – picturing the launch with no audience at all! Although we reached the venue very early people soon started flocking in and my spirits rose. The occasion was also another launch for *Parents* and five contributors including Dilys read from it. The evening went like a dream. Stephen introduced me and I was very touched because he paid such a tribute to me both as a poet and a person. It was wonderful to feel the warm waves of support.

CHAPTER THIRTEEN

Climbing Back to Strength 1

26th October 2000

I managed to revise 'Voicebox' and send it off to the *Scintilla* competition a week before the extended closing date. It's very satisfying to have finished this long poem. At the back of my mind I'm already wondering what I will tackle next. Even though I'll probably want at least two or three years before I develop another narrative I'd like to have the seed of an idea germinating.

It's wonderful to have so much positive feedback about the new books but I'm also experiencing a sense of anti-climax. I think it's because I saw the autumn's publications as a golden prize waiting for me when the ordeal of the treatments was finally over. At some level I think I must have convinced myself that once the books were out I'd no longer be officially ill and that I'd simply pick up something akin to my ordinary life. Now I'm looking at the bald truth: I feel tired almost all the time, quickly become exhausted and am still miles away from the strength I had before the operation. I'm only just beginning to appreciate how much the treatments weakened me. I want to do the 'Writing for Self-Discovery' course at Missenden Abbey next weekend and Erwin has kindly offered to drive me there and collect me afterwards which will make the journey easy. I suppose I am pushing myself a bit but I know I'm capable of doing it so I don't intend to give in. Unfortunately though I can't find any way to turn off my anxiety. It's not just the course – anything and everything seems to worry me at the moment and I'm in and out of panic several times a day. As I said to Mimi on the phone all my faults are exaggerated so that I'm a caricature of myself!

27th October

Note for a poem

Lying in bed last night I began to think about the images of Noah I'd used in the poem about the blind girl in the Chagall Museum. I suppose this was because it was raining yet again, also because I know Noah needs to come out of that poem. It has too much about Chagall's paintings. I found myself picturing Noah as the first environmentalist, saw him in the Ark with the hot stink of fox, the mustard smell of lion and with the animals, birds and insects all settling down. Then I imagined him letting off the dove into a cauldron of light and later, after the floodwaters had subsided, lying on lush grass. Half asleep I visualized a modern Ark full of gadgets, entry being refused to animals. The waters rose and I saw it sailing over city roads and towerblocks. But when this flood subsided there was nothing but wastes of grey mud and no people – just a few shells of buildings, concrete railings and other bits of debris on a planet that was barren, useless as a worn out tennis ball. Then I was standing holding the bald tennis ball in the palm of my hand.

30th October

Adrian Taylor, our aged neighbour, has died. We made a batch of soup for him every week. He was doing quite well in the nursing home which his friend, Pam managed to get him into at the beginning of September. Erwin visited him once a week and heard many stories about his past life. Just over a week ago he had another stroke – I'm glad he didn't linger on, ill and incapacitated. I shall miss him. Every time I make soup or read my poem, 'Soup and Slavery', I shall remember him.

6th November

What I'm calling the 'overwhelm' syndrome got completely out of hand last week. I went on feeling anxious about the Missenden Abbey course even though we'd organized it so that John would take a couple of sessions by himself if I began to flag. The upshot of all this was that for four or five nights beforehand I slept badly. When it came to it though the weekend went very well. I enjoyed being away from home where I've been forced to spend so much of the year. I did feel tired on and off but I managed perfectly well and didn't need to leave John to run any sessions on his own. Someone on the course with a lively prose style had written about very difficult personal experiences and I was able to give her some help in a one-to-one session. I came home feeling much more confident about what I can manage.

In spite of the boost of the weekend I'm still finding this recovery period very uncomfortable. While I was recuperating from the operation and undergoing treatment I frequently felt frightened or upset but rarely depressed. I not only braced myself to go through the ordeal, I clung like a leech to everything life-giving and positive. Now, however, I often feel depressed – as if everything's impossibly hard, as if health and ordinary living are forever out of reach. Any problems throw me completely. Erwin has a painful joint in his big toe – arthritis maybe. Just as I'm feeling ready to go out more he's finding walking hard. There doesn't appear to be any easy or obvious solution. It's as if we're on a permanent downhill. I feel mean for thinking of his foot as a problem that limits me instead of being sympathetic. After all Erwin's given me support for months and months without making a whisper of complaint that I've restricted his life.

8th November

I've told Kate that I'm finding life a terrible struggle at the moment and she's pointed out that I am at a very early stage of recovery and expecting too much of myself emotionally as well as physically. She made me see that this period of re-adjustment really *is* very difficult. She also told me that I am doing very well. It's dawned on me that this feeling of being completely overwhelmed is to be expected and that if I keep blaming myself for managing badly I'm simply giving myself another problem. I felt enormously relieved after this discussion. We also talked about my fear of death. I described how I saw two guns pointing at my head when I was given the diagnosis and how my first thought was: I'll never feel safe again. I believed I'd come to terms with this but Kate said she thought the fear had been displaced and that I was acting it out in any and every anxiety that troubled me. This makes sense. She asked me what I feared about death and I said: 'Losing consciousness. It's a precious gift and it's terrible to lose it.' I also talked about being afraid of life thinned, the pain and weakness of dying. As I write this I can see my fear of death does underlie everything else. I carry a strong feeling, which I know is not unique, that if my poetry is recognized then at least my work will last and in a sense I will not die. Of course I know there can be no guarantee of this. We also talked about taking control of catastrophic fear and other anxieties because being ruled by these is in itself a dimming of consciousness, a kind of death.

Kate suggested meditation with a candle and for some days I've tried sitting – or better – lying down and looking at a lit red candle for five or ten minutes. I've concentrated on the licking flame brightening the red globe with its small determined blade of light, the pale image of a second reflected flame behind it, the wick at its core. I've also imagined the candlelight inside my body, its illumination releasing me from all worry and fear, whatever is on my mind, imagined it filling me with warmth, quiet and calm. 'Looking-at-the-candle' time has also been 'taking-stock' time, a time to switch off the pressures, in particular to stop saying to myself: 'Your illness is over, why aren't you getting on with life, making up for the lost year?' Instead I've tried to look at what is actually happening, to allow the good things, count up what I have done instead of listing what I've failed to do and to feed myself with the colour and warmth of the candle.

I'd drafted 'Climbing' by this time. While I was working on it I kept re-living the walk we did to Beachy Head, re-capturing the elation which I lost during October. I began to understand I was going through a depression I couldn't allow before. The poem was difficult to write partly because I had so much material and partly because I developed it in three-line stanzas which all ended with an '-ing' word, usually a verb. I'm not sure how I hit on this idea but it carries a sense of continuity and this seemed important. John had some criticisms which I dealt with and later, after one of our Sunday workshops, I shortened it. I've refined it again since then but it's still substantially the poem I wrote in November. Here it is:

Climbing

The sun is out, the sea is in, throwing
salt kisses that snap my skin to life
and each step flattens illness. Unblinking,

a herring gull observes us from the shingle.
We gape as a toytown train trundles
to the last stop on the esplanade, see it's bulging

with unsmiling elderly children, then mount
a street queened by a Victorian mansion.
Stopped by a hump of Down, we hover, sniffing

grass, taking stock of the steepness.
And though a flight of stairs still leaves me
breathless, my body is singing, refusing

the road that sneaks off to the left.
Slowly we climb above the white hotels,
the bandstand's curves, the pier perching

on bird stilts, above unfolding swathes
of sea. Clouds scuttle as I spread
my hands across the sky – I'm kicking

seven months of sickness to the cliffs' edge.
Clicking a gate, we're hemmed in
by knobbly hawthorns, by elders dangling

jet clusters beyond our reach. In clefts
and rabbit holes possibilities glint
but they're trapped by stems threatening

to ribbon flesh. Suddenly we're tipped onto
open Down, watch the sun dipping the sea
in turquoise, olive, needled gold, hushing

it to a grey that's paler than hopelessness
as if to ram the point: water wears
many colours, possesses none. Turning,

we gain the ridge, peer at an arm of land
and a new coast: the Seven Sisters,
seven white determined faces, jutting

into a distance which beckons. We walk towards
a glittering spur of Beachy Head. Holes
are gouged in the chalk face and it's hanging

defenceless as a half-demolished house
but unbeaten. In the museum we'll put
names to birds we've seen, ignore the bleatings

of the lifelike shepherd doomed to explain
his life for ever, learn how fossilized shells
banked, grew into walls that belittle buildings,

make insects of humans. Kneeling on turf,
I'm thrummed by air the sun's combed,
by the green running through blades,
the seagull rise of cliff. *I* am not crumbling.

14th November

Kate has given me another visualization to experiment with. The first step is to picture the fear I experienced when I was given the diagnosis and then imagine in precise detail putting it into a box and shutting the lid. The second stage is to take the box and secrete or bury it some-where well away from myself. The last step is to replace the fear with another feeling. I tried this out lying in bed at night – pictured a heavy trunk like the one I used to take to college, stuffing miles of fear into it, banging the lid down, sitting on it to make sure it stayed shut, then fitting the metal clasps and turning its lock. After that I saw myself tipping the trunk into the brook which runs through the park behind our house, waiting while it sank into the stream's muddy bed. Finally I encouraged a sense of calm to grow inside me and permeate my whole body. It's amazing how well this works.

> Since then I've used this exercise and variations of it many times to separate myself from fear or worry. It may sound simplistic or childlike but when I've been distressed I've found it extraordi-narily powerful and satisfying.

16th November

At last I've managed to cope with visiting the dentist for a check-up and to discuss my broken teeth – another hurdle. I explained I didn't feel strong enough to undergo much treatment and was relieved when she decided the broken teeth should wait until January. I'm sure this was the right decision because the work she did do – two small fillings – caused me to wake up in the middle of the following night with toothache. Needless to say I panicked and asked for an emergency appointment but the pain wore off over the next day or two. Normally I see Kate for counselling once a month but we're fitting in some extra sessions and these are giving me more resources. I must admit though I'm still finding life very hard going.

I've started work on 'Flood' using the notes I made about the rain, Noah and my vision of a new flood. I'm haunted by the image of the world shrunk to an over-used tennis ball. I think this poem is a departure for me and it feels good to be writing something that's not personal. I'm allowing it plenty of time to develop.

21st November

Things are slowly moving on. I've done more work with Kate about managing the critical voice in my head which is still banging on: 'You ought…come on…it's your fault…you're no good' etc. We've talked about being kind to myself and allowing my distressing feelings instead of letting that wretched critical voice cut in and urge me to suppress them. I'm missing the regular contact I had with clients and staff at Flightways every week. Possibly I need to replace this with something that takes me out of the house or maybe the adjustment will come about naturally.

26th November

I'm thinking about re-writing the poem about the blind girl in the Chagall Museum. I must make sure the paintings don't compete with the girl. As John commented she didn't even appear until the fourth verse. I realize I felt unsure how to approach her, worried among other things about being sentimental and it was much easier to write about those irresistible paintings. I don't feel such a need to write about them now I've drawn on the Noah painting for the 'Flood' poem. I intend to concentrate on the girl, explore her more fully.

Flow-Writing about the blind girl

She's closed off, apart. Why is she sitting so still in this place where colours leap out? It isn't natural for a child to sit so still. She's folded away in pale elegant grey. Long quiet hair. She's so intent she shifts my attention from Jacob's ladder. All round us the Old Testament figures who dance in our imaginations – their wrestlings, their visions – are out of her reach. Wasn't it cruel to bring her to this place dedicated to sight? Does she tell colour by the smell of daffodils, grass, oranges; know cinnamon from its grains in her hands; taste the gold of honey? Her white face is poignant. Her sore sticky eyes follow me from canvas to canvas. Note: the end of my first attempt – where she's standing close to the painting of Adam and Eve in paradise – feels more or less right.

> The second version of the poem didn't come easily either but it did focus on the blind girl and I was sure it had moved on. There were eight lines about how the girl might sense colour which I both liked and queried because they took the poem in another direction. John thought it was greatly improved. However, I took it to our Sunday workshop a couple of months later and Mimi pointed out that what really worked strongly was the interaction between the girl and the paintings and that my reactions – which had in fact been the most difficult thing to write – stood in the way. I knew at once that she was right but it was another six months before I felt I could work on the material again. Then I was surprised how quickly I produced a much shortened version and I was rather ashamed of the over-writing in the earlier versions. At last I believed the poem worked. Here it is:

In The Chagall Museum

Why is she sitting so small and tightly closed?
Nine at most, her stillness compels, wrests
attention from Jacob on the ladder wrestling with dream.

Curled over the sheaf of white papers on her lap,
mice fingers on row after row of raised dots,
she's marooned in this temple dedicated to sight.

Is she reading about Jacob's braced mauve back,
the silver lick illuminating his knee muscles? Is mauve
to her the honeyed scent of buddleia, taste of brambles?

Angels billow, midnight blues and sensual reds
leap from the walls but don't erase her fluent fingers,
the sticky soreness of her half-shut eyes.

Now she's being guided towards Adam and Eve,
Chagall lovers at ease among lighthearted bouquets
and woolly animals. She's placed at a hand's width

from the wolf, must be looking at its plum pelt
with peripheral vision. Can she see the crouched lion,
the green prancing in the garden? Abruptly she turns away.

Nearby the guilty pair run from garden of paradise
to a world of wrongs. Below them at exactly her height
a purple fish is plunging, flippers spread like wings.

I'm still tired and easily thrown but I don't feel quite as ground down as I did. I went to the London Lapidus meeting yesterday. This organization promotes the value of personal writing. Its members include therapists, writers, creative writing tutors, academics and other people interested in using writing in all its forms for personal development. The meeting was a session to discuss what the London branch should do. I was pleased everyone wanted sessions which would focus on sharing experience and ideas and there was something about spending an afternoon at a meeting which wasn't essential work that made me feel at last I was on my way back to normal life.

CHAPTER FOURTEEN

Climbing Back to Strength 2

28th November 2000

Mice in The Underground: Poem note

At Bond Street station, on the way home from a concert, two mice quite near, circling the empty platform at extraordinary speed. They must have been searching for food but found neither crumb nor crisp. After a bit they disappeared over the platform edge down the sheer side to the rails where they were at risk from the crush of rushing noise. These mice have no way out, have never experienced daylight, never sniffed grass, made nests in walls, holes or hedges. They are like hopeless clockwork toys, switched on until their small mad engines give out or are stopped.

1st December

I've started writing Christmas cards and I realize there are still some people with whom I only have occasional contact who don't know I've had breast cancer this year.

On Wednesday Dilys and I went to a Cats Night Out evening which had a focus on *Parents*. These monthly poetry readings at the

Poetry Café in Covent Garden provide a platform for women poets. They usually feature two poets as well as offering time for floor readings and they're extremely popular. The organizer, poet Angela Dove, has put a great deal of work into Cats Night Out and she is sensitive and insightful in her responses to all the poets who read. On Wednesday *Parents* was featured and she began by praising the anthology warmly. The whole evening was lively and thought-provoking.

On Thursday I gave a tutorial and my sense of returning normality has continued but I still feel tired most of the time and have no reserves to fall back on. For a couple of days I think I'm on top of everything, then I sleep badly or something upsets me and I'm struggling again!

7th December

For the last few days I've been sleeping better but I never seem to get enough rest. I'm slow to focus and I wonder if the Tamoxifen has something to do with this or the depression I still feel on and off. Altogether I'm full of contradictions. On the one hand I need and want plenty of time for writing. On the other hand part of me wishes for a week with more activities built in. I suspect if I had this I'd be worried about losing my writing time. Why can't I just leave things open for the moment and feel pleased I can make changes when I'm ready? Is the real problem that my strength is limited? It's an effort to remember the good things but there are some. I did a reading for Salisbury House Poets in Enfield last Saturday. The evening was well attended and the audience was extremely appreciative and interested in my books. There are more fixtures for next year. And I'm still writing a lot – even I am amazed by my output during the last ten months and John says I've produced some of my strongest poems this year. I do feel that my work is developing yet I'm somehow afraid my health might stop my writing from moving on. This is in spite of the fact that I've used illness as a way of extending my work.

On a more mundane level I'm just beginning to feel I might get some pleasure again from cooking. I suppose it's not surprising that the chemotherapy turned me off food preparation even more than it turned me off food. Yet food is something I've always relished and in the past when not pressed for time I've found cooking nurturing too.

Guns of death: Flow-Writing

The moment I was told I had cancer what I saw were two guns, one perched on each of the consultant's shoulders and their nostrils were pointing straight at me, long nostrils full of death. I wanted to refuse the news, keep it outside my body, outside my mind. Couldn't. The structure of my life collapsed like flimsy overladen furniture and a voice in my head repeated over and over and over in dreadful tones: 'Never, you will never ever feel safe again, never...' This feels like material for a poem.

> I'd written about this, of course, two days after I was given the diagnosis and I'd thought of it now and then during the year. Four weeks previously when Kate asked me to describe the moment to her she'd shown me that I was still reacting to it and I began to see that the shock and the emotions which it triggered were still lodged deep inside me, that I needed to re-record the event in order to begin to come to terms with it. It may still be a poem I want to write. I don't know.

15th December

The continual rain has stopped at last. There's bright sun and the exhilarating sharpness of winter in the air. I love the way red, pink and gold spread over the sky as the sun goes down and how, after it appears to be dark looking out through a window, one can walk down the road into the park and follow the last minutes of light in the luminous blue of the west.

Anne Cluysenaar has written a review of *Insisting on Yellow*. She's made points that particularly pleased me. One of them is: 'Someone has said that the deeper we go in ourselves, the more we come up in other people. These poems frequently evoke the process whereby

self-understanding may lead to acute empathy for others.' The piece
has been printed in the Second Light Newsletter.

20th December

After an interval of nearly six months we started our N7 workshop
again on Sunday – just four of us at the meeting: Mimi, Caroline and
her partner, Clive, and me. I was so glad Mimi managed to come. Afterwards we sat down to the Christmas feast that's become a tradition
after our December meeting. I made a chicken casserole and the others
brought a salad and sweet. I was quite worried by the comments about
my poem which I think needs much more work and I found myself
wilting by the end of the meal but it was lovely to re-start the group,
another tangible sign of returning normality.

On Monday I had a session with Kate. It hit me that I had sunk
back into the same frame of mind as I'd been in at the beginning of the
previous session. In other words my critical voice had leapt out of
control again. It was as if I'd forgotten everything we'd talked about
last time and I'd allowed myself to be ruled yet again by the invisible
but dominating creature which finds fault with everything I do or
don't do. It's so destructive, such a waste of energy. Kate managed to
open a new door for me which I think will enable me to throw off this
critical voice more firmly. I now have a new determination to be on the
lookout and not let it take possession of me. I intend to arrive at the
next counselling session in a more positive state of mind.

23rd December

'Choosing Yellow': More notes

The raucous bill of a toucan I saw in Trinidad's rainforest. Yellow is
winter jasmine, its thin lemon petals hedging the wall; the kitchen
sharp with the sting of lemons; the hard yellow of the oilskins I was
made to wear when I was eight, its scratch on shins and wrist, being
torn to ribbons by the jeer of 'yellow chicken' on the school bus.
Yellow is combs of honey and the body's honey-softness when the

gold embroidery of pain is unpicked, the gloss on yellow peppers, the striped yellow curtains holding off heat's overpowering stare and cold's peck. Yellow is the place where I find present and past woven together, a state of mind, the hope I trawl across shifting sands, the marmalade I put on toast to fortify myself when I can't sleep in the middle of the night – the tangy strips of peel blending with jellied sweetness. Yellow is wild flowers threatened by today's chemicals but struggling to survive: celandine, cowslips, lady's slipper, the dandelions I picked when I was four – not understanding why they drooped. Yellow is a place to hold onto when your world is falling apart for whatever reason, holding on – survival.

3rd January 2001

In the main the Christmas and New Year break has been a pleasant and relaxing change from routine. On Christmas Day we had supper at Ben and Pogle's new house. They've moved the cat in and half moved themselves. On New Year's Eve the usual small gathering of long-standing friends came here. I was so pleased that I had the stamina to cook dinner for nine people and stay up to see 2001 in. I had no idea the first year of the new millennium would be so traumatic and difficult. I hope 2001 will be easier!

7th January

It's now a year since I was recalled by the breast screening clinic – a year that's changed my life. I still feel shocked that I've had cancer – as if death had brushed past me. I'm still shocked too that I've lost such a distinctive and key part of my body. The recovery stage is still a drag: tiredness, a sense of powerlessness, exaggerated reactions. Over the holiday period I managed most of the time to hang onto myself and not let that pushy critical voice take over. Now and then I have the sense of emerging from a very long tunnel.

I've got over another hurdle: my broken teeth – one is going to be crowned, the other filled. On Thursday the root canal and main drilling work was done. I've been trying to work out why I'd built up such a mountain of worry about this. I think the memory of a complication when I had a tooth crowned a couple of years ago was exaggerated by all I've been through. Anyway the long session at the dentist's went much more easily than I expected and I noticed how much stronger I felt than I did when I went for a check-up in November. There was hardly any discomfort afterwards.

8th January

In the park the copse is where I most feel the presence of nature and a sense of otherness, the unexplained, the spiritual. The trees are mainly oaks but there are also hawthorns, elderberry, holly trees, a few firs and beeches which grow from a cluster of trunks. Where do roots end and stems begin? It's not struck me before how they run into one another. Some trunks look very rootlike as they emerge from the ground and the knobbled roots at the base of large trees seem like extensions of the trunk. I've heard the woodpecker drilling branches in this copse and when we're having a walk at dusk or in the dark we often hear the hollow cries of owls, those voices of elsewhere going on and on as if fixated. I love the nutty smells of leaves and leaf mould, the sweet tartness of brambles, also the layers of darkness beneath trees, like the different layers of self.

11th January

The writing workshops have started again and people are saying how much better I am looking than I did five weeks ago. I am very aware now of moving forward. It's a nuisance that I'm still having trouble with sleeping but I've always found switching off when I go to bed a problem so it's hardly surprising it's been worse during the last year. I often go through the visualization of shutting up nagging worries in a box and then shutting the box away. This has a very calming effect.

It took me a while to see how to develop the 'yellow' notes. There were too many flower references and I cut out van Gogh – he's been

over-used by poets. A poem started to gel once I'd decided to follow
trains of thought and melt one image into the next – the fluidity
seemed crucial. Once I'd hit on the idea of breaking the line each time
the thought shifted and worked out a route for these shifts, the
drafting was comparatively easy. I was far on in this when I saw how
important the survival idea is and I now realize survival has been key
in most of the new ideas I've had in the last three months whatever the
subject. This is bound to be a theme in my next collection of poetry.
John and Caroline are both enthusiastic about this poem.

Choosing Yellow
for Les

Because I've insisted on yellow you write saying
Porsche yellow's your favourite, define it as the buttercup
of Hohenzollern blended with Habsburg's rich
egg yolk, want to know which shade I prefer.
Immediately I see
               my child self plunging
hands into dandelion ranks bugling brightness
from a dirt pavement, see my paint brush laden
with nectar from a cowslip cube, filling outlines
of fairytale caskets
             the petals we sold as butter
on the paint-needy bench by the barbed
wire field opposite our house while far below
the great grey slugs of warships sat motionless
on the Clyde's highway.
               An echo of that colour
on my kitchen cupboards which like the past
are always clicking open. It's stronger

than the lemon
                    I've seen infiltrating hard
green fruits in Andalusian orchards, quieter
than the skin of the plump lemon that's sitting
in my larder. When I cut slices its zest
stings my nicked finger,

                              resurrects the curtains
with uneven hems I made years ago
to keep the kitchen from heat's stare, from cold
feathered with frost. Winter pecking at flesh
summons up

                    that unyielding oilskin with a hood
my mother made me wear whenever it rained,
not knowing I was torn to ribbons on the school bus
by the hot pack chanting: *yellow chicken.*
The shameful label, still stitched to my body,
jumps me to a badge

                        I've only seen in black
and white photographs: the star Hitler forced
other Jews to wear…

                    Yellow is the percussion
of light beneath clouds heavy as persecution,
the sweetness running from waxy cells, the body
soft as fur when pain's sharp gold embroidery
is unpicked.

                    It sings from the bumble-bee slash
on a motorway truck, wild flowers massed
on grass: celandine, lady's slipper, tormentil,
tiny warriors pitting themselves against
air fogged with chemicals…

                You see I can't extract
a single yellow. It's a bittersweet colour
which feeds emptiness in the middle of the night,
a state of mind that refuses fear. It's any place:
thistle field, ditch, shore with shifting sand
where hope survives.

18th January

I've been thinking about the way my body's been healing itself silently, gradually without conscious participation of my mind, how it's withstood shock, mutilation, stood up and fought back against the powerful treatments that have damaged it. For the first time maybe I see my body as a separate force carrying out its own purposes although it and I are inextricable, always influencing one another. But as my awareness of recovery increases I can sit here writing and contemplate this with wonder.

I'm delighted that *Acumen* magazine has accepted Anne's essay about *Insisting on Yellow* and I now have a date for my reading at the Ledbury Poetry Festival. The amazingly energetic and dedicated Barbara Large has been in touch with me about this year's Writers' Conference at King Alfred's College in Winchester at the end of June. I've agreed to run a workshop and give a talk. 2001 is going to be busy!

26th January

It's almost a year since the diagnosis and I feel it's time to bring my cancer journal to an end, to let my notebook revert to being a place in the main for writing ideas. In the last couple of weeks I've been conscious of having more energy. I can just about manage a full morning's writing and although I am still some distance from my full strength I'm something akin to what I think of as myself. I feel readier to accept that my energy can only return slowly and I feel more grounded.

I had no idea that the entry I made in my notebook on 12th January last year was the beginning of a journal. During the last thirteen months I've often lost confidence and felt hopelessly dependent on Erwin. At the same time the illness has taken me into a new dimension and made me value life, its preciousness more than I've ever done before. I also believe I have found a new inner strength, a new assertiveness, a new capacity to persist. I've been carried by the kindness and compassion I've received from Erwin, Ben, my closest friends, many other friends, doctors, nurses and people I only know slightly. I have always found writing supportive, believed that it crystallizes and validates experience. Never have I found it more powerful than in the last year. Writing has taken me into new areas of creativity and helped me to carry out my determination to live every moment of my life as fully as I can.

Afterword

26th July 2002

It is nearly two years now since I finished the chemotherapy. This book has been written and also most of the poems I want to put into my next collection of poetry. I have continued to gain strength. In fact I think I am still gaining strength. Every three months I have a check-up. I am, of course, very pleased that I am being carefully monitored but I am always tense beforehand, afraid that a new tumour will be discovered. At first I was extremely ashamed of these fears but now I know others experience similar feelings and recognize that they are very understandable.

On a cold night in February last year Dilys and I were in Durham for the northern launch of *Parents*. Anne Stevenson introduced the book and read her marvellous poem, 'Arioso Dolente', which is in the anthology. Contributors from Durham, Northumberland and Yorkshire also read their poems. In March I heard that my narrative poem, 'Voicebox', had won the first prize in the long poem section of the *Scintilla* poetry competition. I was elated. It seemed like another way of defeating cancer. In June I ran a four-day writing workshop in Penzance and did a reading. I also tutored workshops and gave readings in other parts of the country. During my travels I met two women who had had a recurrence of breast cancer but had come through and were living full lives. I felt reassured by their survival and admired their no fuss attitude, their resilience.

Last September I gave a talk to London Lapidus about the ways in which writing had supported me during my illness. This April I had the extraordinary and exhilarating experience of speaking about 'Writing Poetry in Extremity' with some reference to the work of Henry Vaughan to a roomful of poets and professors at The Colloquium of Usk Valley Vaughan Association. In preparing the talk I found it illuminating to consider how extreme situations generate creativity and to read in more detail the work of this metaphysical poet who wrote many of his powerful and visionary poems at a time of extremity in his life.

Since last summer three women I know have been diagnosed with breast cancer and been in touch with me. Sharing the experience of the cancer with others who have been diagnosed with it, hearing and passing on that it is possible to come through and even to make something out of the illness, is very sustaining.

PART II

Writing Ideas

Introduction

You may want to keep a journal to chart your journey through illness. When life is stressful, writing about what you are going through might be very supportive, more helpful at times than looking for ways to escape. It can help you sort out your reactions and make sense of the experience. You may find, like me, that your diary or notebook is invaluable as a place to release chaotic feelings and work out how best to cope with what lies ahead, also a place to record ideas and moments of enjoyment. The writing suggestions which follow are almost all ones I used in my journal and I hope they will offer some possibilities you would like to try out.

On the other hand you might feel that keeping a continuous record, even if you only add to it now and then, would be tiresome or too much of a pressure – given everything else on your plate. You might prefer the thought of writing only when you have had a strong reaction to something, when you're feeling buoyed up or very low or simply when you feel in the mood to write. It may suit you to work your way through the different approaches I suggest or you may prefer to pick out the ideas which most appeal to you. You will probably find that some of the techniques work better for you than others.

When you write try and do it with a biro or pen that runs easily. I think it's best to write in an exercise book or writing pad – maybe something with an attractive cover. If you use sheets or scraps of paper keep them together in a folder. It's possible that you'll want to look at some of your pieces of writing again and that you'll find they offer insights or suggest other subjects you want to explore. There may be pieces you'd like to develop further or use as starting points for poems. Most importantly I believe you will find writing supportive and affirming. When I wrote about matters outside myself I felt alive and involved. When I poured out my anxieties and fears I was almost always aware of a lightening. Sometimes I was uplifted by a new idea or insight. Very occasionally you may find you need to continue writing or do another piece of writing to resolve or calm difficult thoughts and feelings. If this does not seem sufficient then it is a good idea to talk over what's on your mind with someone you are close to or possibly to seek professional counselling.

When you sit down to do some writing try and choose a place where you feel comfortable. It may be at a table in a quiet room – or a noisy one if that's your taste – on an easy chair, your bed or a fleecy rug. Of course, write at a word processor or on the computer if that's what you feel most at home with. I often wrote on the tube when I went for treatment. This was partly because I like writing on trains – the sense of being carried forward seems to go with generating words and ideas – and partly because it completely separated me from the chemotherapy or radiotherapy session which lay ahead.

Starting Off

1. At this moment

This is a good way to start writing under any circumstances and is particularly useful if you don't know where to begin; if you are feeling upset and worried; if your head is spinning with a jumble of incidents, people, discomforts, conflicting thoughts and feelings. First of all describe in some detail anything which catches your attention. It might be a headline on the newspaper crumpled on the floor, a thoughtful or amusing card someone's sent you, sunlight coming through smeared windows, a cup of tea with steam coming off it, a picture on the wall, a scarf, light catching on a bottle, car keys, a tree you can see outside. If you prefer pick something you've done, heard or thought today – something which is easy to write about and not one of your main preoccupations. Spend up to ten minutes on this but five minutes or less if you're feeling anxious about putting pen to paper.

Now move on to writing about what is on your mind at the moment. Don't worry whether you are doing it well or correctly. This writing is for you – at this stage anyway – and whatever you note down will be right for you. If you want to bring in all kinds of details, problems and feelings without explaining them, then do so. Feel free to be as irrational, fearful, angry, uncertain, repetitive as you like. If you find yourself exploding in single words, writing rambling notes or images, that's fine. If you find you want to concentrate on people or incidents or something which doesn't relate closely to you at all, that's fine too.

My entry for 12th January in Chapter One is an 'At this moment' piece. I ran a writing workshop that evening and we began the session with this exercise which I did too. Something prompted me to write my piece in my notebook for writing ideas and not on a piece of paper as I usually do in workshops. I wasn't thinking of keeping a journal at that point but I remember that I felt the need to record what was happening and to release my feelings. I began by describing waking up in the morning and this led naturally into what was on my mind. (For this book I cut out some of the repetitions in the piece and added some outer detail so that readers would be able to follow my train of thought.)

2. High moments and low moments

During a serious illness it's not surprising if one has extreme reactions. I often found myself overwhelmed by fear or trapped in anxiety. When this occurred everything else seemed to disappear. I found though that writing about high and low moments helped me to hang on to the good things I experienced as well as giving me space to express my feelings about the bad ones. I would recommend writing about high and low moments and setting the pieces side by side to create a balanced picture.

(a) Begin by writing down five high moments from the last few days. By high moments I mean anything that you've enjoyed, found comforting, interesting, anything that's given you an insight or taken you away from worry and/or discomfort. High moments are likely to arise from quite small occurrences, for example: an illuminating conversation, looking at a child's drawings, a friend's kindness or having a drink with a friend, being warmed by a bowl of soup, stroking a cat, being hugged, being taken out of oneself by a film or television documentary, laughing aloud about something ridiculous, a new and positive perception of your illness, listening to music. In the few days after my operation some of the high moments I wrote about were the surprise of seeing Vicki (6th February, Chapter Three) and the comforting bath I had (8/9th February). Choose one of the high moments you've noted down and write a paragraph about it. Try to re-live it and pinpoint what moved, excited or pleased you.

(b) Jot down four low moments from the last few days. These might be major or minor. My low moments in the few days after I came home from hospital included feeling unable to cope in the middle of my first night at home (13th February, Chapter Four), the fear I felt after the breast cancer nurse gave me some information about chemotherapy (16th February) and the hour and a half Erwin spent searching for his credit card (18th February). Choose a low moment from your list and write as much as you want to about it.

(c) Try making some connections between high and low moments. After she'd had a mastectomy Mary MacRae wrote in her notebook while she was still in hospital:

> Walking up and down the corridor just now I thought that all this was like an endurance test, a kind of difficult exam that I very much wanted to pass.

I would see this as a high moment because it offered her a positive approach, a way of coping. Interestingly the exam idea, potent for her as a teacher, offered her a way a little later on to write a poem about the low moment when she received the diagnosis:

Appointment
by Mary MacRae

The day I kept the first appointment
a large black crow in a tree
cawed as I walked out of the car park –
a clichéd augury.

It only took an hour to tell me
what I didn't know –
the one exam I've ever failed –
a cruel hammer-blow.

When I came out the day had slipped,
the light was out of gear,
something rhymed which shouldn't have done,
I shrugged away a stare

and hurried on; under a lamp
I saw my shadow grow,
overtake me, stretch ahead
as black as any crow.

The notebook entry gave Mary a new view of herself, enabled her to write about her sense of shock and defeat about 'the one exam I've ever failed' in the knowledge that she had moved beyond this stage and that her future had opened up again. Although the poem itself offers no solutions it helped her to begin assimilating the trauma she had been through.

Look through your high moments again and see if there is one which helped you deal in some way with a low moment. Write a few sentences about this.

Letting Go in Lists

List-making might sound like a boring activity which has as much to do with real writing as producing a shopping list. However, the kind of list-making I'm about to suggest is very potent. I used it a number of times and it always had a remarkable effect on my feelings. At a time when one is physically weak this technique has the added advantage that it doesn't require much writing.

1. Dumping

If I was feeling shocked, frightened or in turmoil I found this the most helpful technique of all. I would suggest it as a technique to resort to at any time that you feel upset, can't imagine how you'll get through or sort things out. Sit down, if possible in a place where you are not likely to be disturbed, and make a list of all the feelings and thoughts on your mind. My experience is that this works best if:

(a) You put down each thing that occurs to you as a single sentence.

(b) Start each sentence on a new line.

(c) Write your sentences or most of them in a very simple pattern. This might be: 'I am…', 'I am feeling…', 'I am afraid…', 'I want…', 'I don't want…', 'I don't know…', 'I'm upset because…' etc. For example:

> I am afraid of being very weak and muzzy.
>
> I am afraid of not being in control.
>
> I am afraid of being seen as a feeble coward.

This is from the dumping list I wrote the night before I had my mastectomy. Using a repeated opening helps carry you along. It also gives a poem-like pattern which will underline your mood. Don't worry if some of the sentences don't fit into the pattern and feel free to change the pattern as the list proceeds. My 'I am afraid' changed to 'I want' towards the end of the list above. Don't feel you ought to explain anything or sort anything out. Try to write whatever suggests itself however vague, ridiculous or muddled it seems and allow yourself to write whatever words come into your mind. The items on your list might be panicky, crazily angry, full of swearing, sad, fanciful, self-pitying, mocking, foolish, outrageous. It doesn't matter. They express what is going on inside you. Nobody else has to see what you've written unless you want them to. Your notebook or piece of paper is a place where you can feel safe and free to write, to dump absolutely anything you need to.

When I used this technique on the night before my operation I had an enormous sense of release. My dread of the next morning was hugely reduced – I even felt a sense of elation. It wasn't just that I'd clarified my feelings, I was aware of physically lifting them and placing them outside myself. There they were in tangible words in my notebook and contained in a way that wasn't possible when they were rushing around inside my head. Every time I let go in this way my mood became much more positive even on occasions when my feelings remained mixed. (See 4th February, Chapter Two for the whole of the list quoted above; and 17th February, Chapter Four, 27th February, Chapter Five for other dumping lists.)

2. Taking stock

This technique offers another way of exploring what's happening to you. It's more deliberate than dumping but I found it helpful as a way of assimilating and assessing where I was at. It can offer useful pointers too about what you find most supportive and maybe need more of. It can also help you to pinpoint exactly what is troubling you or what is worrying you most and this might be a first step in finding a way to face or case a problem.

(a) Make a list of everything you've found supportive in the last two days. Be sure to note down things as simple as ordering a jazzy jumper from a catalogue, tracking down some information on the Internet, a neighbour you hardly know dropping in and offering help, a child making you laugh or offering you a cup of tea, reading a chapter in a good book, losing yourself in a love story in a magazine, finding you are strong enough to nip out and buy new slippers or looking at a splash of colour made by flowers. And make sure you do include everything even if it's only a joke in the newspaper, or a silly comedy sitcom on TV. Your list might also include the support of someone close to you and/or giving help or sympathy to someone else – a teenager or child at home who needs your attention or a friend with a problem.

(b) Now make a list of everything – big or little – that has been difficult in the last two days, e.g. worrying about what lies ahead, not sleeping well, physical discomfort, feeling cut off from normal life, feeling lonely, feeling fed up about cancelling an arrangement, being given advice you find disturbing, an argument with someone in the family, the serious problems of someone you are close to, the washing machine leaking, a row with your teenage daughter, protecting your eight-year-old from your anxiety, the cat bringing in a half-dead bird, feeling let down by a friend who hasn't got in touch, etc.

(c) Look at your two lists and make a third list of things you could realistically do to lessen the strain you are under, make life fuller, more relaxed. This might include all kinds of small changes: making more phone calls to friends, not talking on the phone late in the evening, deciding not to have contact with an acquaintance who adds to your anxiety, making sure you have a walk every day, talking to a cancer helpline, joining a cancer support group, getting out a bit more, asking your partner to do some cooking, expressing appreciation of the support someone close has given you, postponing or cancelling work which you know will exhaust you, arranging to have a massage, making sure you have rest times every day, accepting friends' help with children, shopping, etc.

You might find it helpful to look back at your lists every now and then and see if you want to add anything to them, particularly to the third list. On 2nd March (Chapter Five) I made a list of my main resources as I saw them four weeks after my operation. I didn't note down that Erwin was my main support. I much appreciated all he did for me every day and I wish I'd thought to include his help and kindness on the list.

Flow-Writing

Flow-Writing allows us to go beyond the conscious and tap into feelings, images and ideas below the surface. It invites us to put aside the evaluating, organizing and censuring we are conditioned to use when we write and simply allow ourselves to associate freely – that is to put down the first words that come into our heads, then write down what these make us think of and keep following the train of thought. If we do this some of our deepest feelings and thoughts begin to surface. Flow-Writing is therefore an extraordinarily useful technique for getting to the centre of ourselves and for generating creative writing. When you try out Flow-Writing don't worry if you find yourself producing muddled or trivial material. What appears to be confused or insignificant will lead you to key subject matter if you allow it. It becomes much easier to do with practice so even if you find yourself panicking, write whatever is in your head and keep going. However, to begin with keep your Flow-Writing session short, no more than five or six minutes. As you gain confidence you will probably find yourself wanting to extend some of the sessions.

1. Start by writing the first sentence that comes into your head about something you've noticed today. This could be a news item, a friend's letter, police sirens, buds on a plant, someone frowning, the way the settee's faded, a broken toy, the curve of an ornament, junk mail you

haven't bothered to open, a table that needs clearing, how relaxed your sleeping dog looks, etc. Once you've noted down a sentence continue writing whatever comes into your head for five minutes. If you dry up repeat the last two or three words until something new crops up. The piece I wrote in my notebook about the snowdrops (2nd February, Chapter Two) is a short example of Flow-Writing. This stays quite close to its starting point but you may well travel a long way from where you started.

2.   Now write down (a) the first colour you think of, (b) the first vegetable or fruit you think of, (c) the first sound you think of, (d) the first feeling or state of mind you think of. Using at least two of your chosen words, put down the first sentence that comes into your head. Now Flow-Write, again for five minutes, longer if you feel like it. When you stop underline any sentences, phrases or words which interest you or touch on something important. If you feel like it use one of your underlined sentences or phrases as a starting point either for another Flow-Writing session or for a more deliberate piece of writing. Here is part of a piece of Flow-Writing I did three months after I had stopped writing a journal and gone back to using my notebook as a place to record writing ideas. The starting point was looking at purple grapes in the middle of the night.

> The grapes could be made of dark glass and perhaps purple is my favourite colour. Even though it's the middle of the night light is catching on their skins so they scintillate among the dull canisters in the larder. Each grape is an exuberant wink, a blink of sun, a capsule of blood. They speak abundance, living – they speak against death. They say: let go of strings, fixtures, musts. Purple grapes mean Keats' 'Ode to a Nightingale' and the pull between life and death. But these grapes say, and I want them to say: pull the moment into your mouth, laugh, eat it – and there's that easygoing man I saw in a radio studio, the way he leant back in his chair while a girl dropped grapes into his mouth one by one.

3. Try using a picture as a starting point. This could be one hanging up in your home or a reproduction in a book or an art postcard. If you prefer use a photograph in a newspaper or book or one you've taken yourself. Write down three sentences about the painting/photograph. Then move into Flow-Writing and continue for seven minutes or longer. The painting may have a strong influence on what you write or it might set off a train of thought which takes you elsewhere. My short notes about 'The Shell' on 10th March (Chapter Five) and the longer note triggered by *The White Iris* on March 19th (Chapter Six) are Flow-Writing.

4. Choose a feeling, subject or problem that you'd like to explore in writing. Put it down as a heading. Write the first sentence about it that comes into your head and again continue writing whatever suggests itself for five minutes or longer. I looked at feelings I'd dumped and used one of these as a starting point for Flow-Writing on 27th February (Chapter Five). My notes for an angry poem on 9th May (Chapter Eight) are also Flow-Writing.

   The more this technique is practised the easier it becomes to let go and 'flow' and the more fruitful it becomes. However, don't be disconcerted if some Flow-Writing sessions produce much more interesting material than others. You might feel it is worthwhile to do a Flow-Writing session for several days in succession both at times when you feel an urge to write and when you feel blank. At times when my thoughts and feelings have been in flux I've found Flow-Writing very potent. I often use it when I'm developing poems and I know other poets do as well. (For more ideas about Flow-Writing and other examples see the book *Writing for Self-Discovery* which I wrote with John Killick.)

Visualizations

Writing about your reactions to illness and other ordeals, as this book illustrates, can be very helpful. Crystallizing feelings in words and the physical action of writing these down is a release. In addition writing helps clarify problems and often lessens anxiety. It is also therapeutic to put illness aside for a while, to be absorbed in different sensations, images, feelings, ideas. Of course if you are stuck at home, on your own a lot, going through debilitating treatment, have other issues to deal with like taking time off work, money worries, a family member with a different health problem or other problem, a relationship that has recently broken up, the care of children and protecting them from your anxiety about your illness, it is extremely difficult to step outside immediate preoccupations. Nevertheless I think it is very valuable to do so if you possibly can even for a short time. Visualizations can be a route to this freedom and writing is one way of using this technique. Sometimes too, visualizations can provide an image for a frightening or upsetting feeling and in doing so help one begin to cope with it.

During the period of my illness and in the recovery period afterwards I found visualizations helped me shift my state of mind when I was feeling weak or miserable or if I couldn't sleep at night. I also found it productive to write about visualizations. Sometimes I did the visualization first and then re-created it and my feelings in a paragraph or two. On other occasions I developed my visualization in writing. I suggest you try out both methods. In some cases you may find writing is all you want to do, in others you may find trying out the visualization without doing any writing is sufficient for you. I am listing a number of different ideas and hope you will enjoy some of them.

1. Visualizations which focus on real places, activities, objects

(a) Picture yourself in an indoor place you find comforting and restful. It might be a colourful kitchen in a friend's house, a pub you sometimes visit, a particular room or niche in your own house, a garden hut, a café, a bookshop, library, a room with an open fire in a cottage, lying on a sofa listening to CDs, etc. Imagine yourself in your chosen place as fully as possible. Focus on the features which give it its character. Think too about some of these things: textures, colours, shapes, the amount of light, sounds you can hear, anything you can smell, what you are doing in this place. Include any feelings or thoughts that come up. The beginning of my first entry in the book on 12th January (Chapter One) is a visualization of myself in bed in the morning. In *44½ Choices you can make if you have cancer*, written by my friends Sheila Dainow, Vicki Golding and Joanna Wright, they recommend using visualizations to help counter frightening feelings and stress. Vicki quotes from her diary:

> I felt very tense and a friend suggested I thought of a place where I'd been really happy and encouraged me to create the image in my mind. It helped me relax my muscles and I felt less tense. I can still see the scene in my mind.

(b) Picture yourself in a landscape or old building you know: on a beach or cliff, in a field, wood, an old church, among castle ruins, by a brook, river or waterfall, on a hill, a mountain, a small island, etc. Again re-create the place in as much detail as possible including sounds, smells, textures, how light or dark it is, the weather and the feelings and associations that come up. My entry for 3rd August (Chapter

Eleven) includes a visualization of the Anglo-Saxon church at Deerhurst.

(c) Now use the same technique to re-live an activity you enjoy: dancing, swimming, walking, playing tennis, playing a musical instrument, rock climbing, going to the theatre, painting, playing with children, cuddling or making love, dressmaking, shopping, having a bath, gardening, driving on an open road, etc. The beginning of my poem 'Bath' (9th March, Chapter Five) is a visualization and one of the things I remember about writing that poem is that it gave me an extraordinary sense of comfort and freedom.

(d) Think about an object you've enjoyed looking at and maybe touching or smelling. It could be a scarf, a fruit, a lavender bag, a hot water bottle in a fleecy cover, a plant, a piece of pottery, a stone, a shell, a carved wooden bowl, etc. If it's feasible I suggest you begin by looking at and touching your chosen object. Then put it aside and picture it as clearly as you can, maybe with your eyes closed. Concentrate on its shape, size, colour, texture, weight, smell. Describe the object – look at it again if you want to – picking out the details you like most. Now focus on the effect the object has on you. What does your object make you think of? My poem about the camellias (28th May, Chapter Nine) and my note about the lavender bag (4th July, Chapter Ten) are both visualizations and the poem 'Lavender' (18th July, Chapter Eleven) takes the lavender visualization further.

(e) Now picture a person who is important to you in some way or, if you prefer, a pet or even a particular kind of animal you like. Write about the person or animal you've chosen as fully as you can. Include character, voice, mannerisms and habits as well as appearance. Then write about the effect he/she/it has on you.

2. Visualizations that draw on the imaginary

These visualizations give you the freedom to draw widely on your imagination and to enjoy playing with images.

(a) Imagine yourself in a fantasy place or landscape or choose a painting or photograph of a scene which appeals to you and imagine yourself in it. You could also begin by listening to music or a tape of bird song, the sound of the sea, etc. Visualize your fantasy place as fully as possible. In addition to its main features you might want to bring in some of these: sounds you can hear, the sky, the light or darkness, the weather, what you can smell, details about trees and plants, animals, birds, insects, fences, walls, stones, the earth, the shore, buildings, etc. Now focus on the effect your fantasy place has on you. My notes about Georgia O'Keeffe's paintings 'The Shell' (10th March, Chapter Five) and 'The White Iris' (19th March, Chapter Six) are visualizations of fantasy landscapes as well as being Flow-Writing. The poem 'The Shell' (17th March, Chapter Six) and 'Elsewhere' (28th March, Chapter Six) have taken the visualizations further.

(b) Imagine your partner, friends, family members or relatives you feel close to – anyone you have found supportive such as a nurse, a neighbour, a friendly shop assistant, a colleague at work, etc., standing near you. Now see these people in two lines facing each other, their hands linked across the gap to create a bed of arms for you to lie on. Picture yourself lying on the bed of arms and allow it to take your weight. Let yourself relax and feel the strength and caring of the people supporting you as it flows into your body. Describe this and the effect it has on you. I used this visualization quite often during my illness and it gave me a feeling of security and great comfort.

(c) Find a small box which intrigues or attracts you. Look at it carefully and imagine that it contains something special. Describe the box and what it might contain. Now picture yourself opening it and finding inside it something magical and/or moving. This could be a ring, a letter, a seashell, a beautiful paperweight, stone, strange coin, historical object, etc. Because this is fantasy it could, if you prefer, contain something too big to fit into a box or maybe an abstract idea like peace, clarity or warmth. Write about the contents of the box and its effect on you. This is a very satisfying visualization which I have tried out myself and in writing workshops including workshops with young children who have no problem giving their imaginations a free rein!

3. Visualizations which focus on healing

The visualizations I've described so far I experienced as supportive, relaxing and enjoyable. I found the ones in this last set had a specific healing effect. I used the first three when I felt exhausted, over-whelmed or knotted up in both mind and body. The last two I found very sustaining when my body was weak and/or my thoughts were troubled. Some of these visualizations turned out to be the starting points of poems. It is probably a good idea to try out these techniques before you write about them but experiment and see what works best for you.

(a) Light a candle and put it in a safe place in a room where you won't be disturbed for a little while. This exercise is very effective in the dark but it works perfectly well in the daytime or with the light on if you prefer this. Sit somewhere comfortable or propped up in bed so that you can see the candle. Give yourself about eight to ten minutes to look at it. It's best to set a timer. Think of this activity as a time to switch off from worry, weakness, anything preoccupying you and concentrate as much as you can on the candle flame: its colour, lumi-nosity, movement. If you find disturbing thoughts creeping in focus on something positive in your life and then return to concentrating on the candle. After a while imagine taking the candlelight inside yourself, think of it calming you, illuminating what's going through your mind. I wrote about trying out this visualization on 8th November (Chapter Thirteen). It could also be done with a bottle in which coloured liquids rise and fall, a glass paperweight or other objects which catch the light.

(b) Choose a beautiful colour. Imagine it rising from your heart to the top of your head and then flowing downwards filling and relaxing each part of your body: the crown of your head, your forehead, eyes, cheeks, ears, jaws, throat, neck, shoulders, arms, hands, fingers, chest, stomach, abdomen, knees, calves, and feet. Now imagine you are floating on an air cushion or magic carpet of the same colour. The air cushion is not only taking your weight, it is absorbing anything which is worrying you. You are released. What colours or thoughts come into your freed mind? I find this technique very calming and writing about it can produce a similar effect. It is a variation of part of 'The Egg of Protection', a relaxation technique on Kate Williams MacKenzie's tape: 'Relaxation and Self-Healing' (see 13th February, Chapter Four). The poem I wrote about the camellias (see 28th May, Chapter Nine) also draws on this visualization.

(c) I found this technique very helpful when I was recovering from my mastectomy. It is one which Kate Williams Mackenzie, my therapist, told me about. Close your eyes and picture the wound or the weak part of your body. Now imagine you are seeing the area through a softening lens and quieten it, blur its edges and whole appearance so that it's less disturbing to look at. Now picture the area being healed by bands of coloured light or words or music or the flow of soothing water, or the feel of creamy lotion, moss, silk, etc. (see 2nd March, Chapter Five).

(d) This visualization is particularly good for stopping a specific worry, fear or other destructive feeling from going round and round in your head and dominating your thoughts. Imagine some shape or form for the feeling or problem that's on your mind: hammers, tangled ropes, nails, skewers, a rock or stones, muffling layers of cloth, etc. Now see yourself shutting the object you've pictured into a box, trunk or chest. Visualize the container you've chosen in detail: its size, shape, colour, what it's made of, how it shuts and see yourself pushing the physical form of the feeling or problem inside, shutting it, maybe locking it or tying it up with string or cord. Now imagine yourself getting rid of the container: dumping it in a river or the sea, locking it away in a cupboard, burying it in the ground or in a cave. Picture this in detail too. Finally replace what you've put in the box with a feeling you would like to experience: calm, acceptance, relaxation, hope, affection, etc. I found this technique, another offered to me by Kate, particularly helpful in the recovery period after my treatment was finished and writing about it in my notebook reinforced its effect (see 14th November, Chapter Thirteen). I still turn to this visualization sometimes if I feel stressed.

In one of the poems in her sequence about cancer, 'Changing The Subject', Carole Satyamurti creates a room which is an image for her ominous feelings. She then replaces it with another room which is the same colour as the first but has features which completely change her state of mind. In the final short verse she moves on to a new viewpoint. I find this poem very moving and see it as a variation of the visualization I've just described. You might like to try it out. You could write about two different rooms or else choose an image of your own as a vehicle for your feelings.

Choosing the Furniture
by Carol Satyamurti

The curtains said:
what do you fear more than anything?
Look at it now.

A white room.
I lie and cannot speak,
can not get up.
I stream with pain from every part.
I cry, scream until the sound chokes me.

Someone at the door looks in,
glances at her watch, moves on.
No one comes. No one
will ever come.

The lamp said:
think of what would be most blissful
– what do you see?

A white room
lined with books; a window
looking out on trees and water;
bright rugs, a couch, a huge table
where I sit, words spinning from my fingers.
No one comes; time is limitless,
alone is perfect.
Someones leaves food at the gate
–fruit, bread, little chocolate birds.

The moon laughed:
there is only one room.
You choose the furniture.

(e) Chemotherapy and radiotherapy destroy cancerous cells but of course
they also attack the healthy body. The body fights back but there may
well be times when treatment makes it very weak. I read in a brochure
that it was therapeutic to imagine the white cells asserting themselves
and combating the attack made on them. During the six months I
underwent treatment, especially when I was lying down having a rest
or if I woke in the middle of the night, I found it calming, enjoyable
and encouraging to conjure up different images of the white cells
rousing themselves. Try this lying down if you feel tired. Let a
vigorous or appealing image which you would like to stand for your
white cells taking action come into your mind. This could be

whacking a kettle drum, a prowling tiger, giant feet trampling, sauce-pans clattering, a troupe of dancers, an army marching, a crane lifting machinery, eight oarswomen or men rowing a boat, runners in a marathon, trumpets trumpeting, fireworks shooting into the sky, etc. Use any of these images or think up your own. Writing might help you conjure up this visualization or be a very satisfying way of reinforcing it. If the idea appeals you could also draw your visualization with coloured pens or pencils and make this a starting point for writing. For me this technique of picturing the white cells was a resource, almost a routine. I often turned to it just for a minute or two when I wasn't up to doing anything else. One of my favourite images was the corps de ballet in Swan Lake: lines of white legs and feet in satin ballet shoes rising in unison in the moonlight. Another, I have no idea why, was gondolas gliding down canals in Venice (see 25th April, Chapter Eight).

Before her first session of chemotherapy poet Alicia Stubbersfield had hypnotherapy which gave her a set of healing images. She wrote in her notebook:

> The session was wonderful. I have a safe place to go. I count five stone steps down into the garden of my childhood with the trees in blossom and the flat sandy stone where the frog lived. I walk round the garden. In chemotherapy my body will be filled with golden healing energy – my white blood cells are like sequins, gleaming as they search out any cancer cells and destroying them. My body is a house and I can switch off nausea like a light.

She told me: 'I remember using the idea of "switching off" the nausea and conjuring up the garden image when I was feeling particularly bad – as a relaxation method.' Hypnotherapy might be something worth exploring if you have the opportunity. Another possibility would be to create for yourself in writing – maybe while listening to music or looking at a painting – images that would offer you a place 'to go' during or after chemotherapy.

Writing About Memories

Trauma and stress are disorientating. Your illness has probably disrupted your life at least for a while and there may be times when you feel weak, isolated, uncertain, stressed, depressed, powerless, and when it's a struggle to hold onto your image of the person you were before your illness. A good way of freeing yourself from your present situation, while at the same time staying with yourself, is to write about your past which is still key to who you are now. Relating yourself to your earlier life can be grounding and affirming. I have just quoted in Visualizations what Alicia Stubbersfield wrote about the garden of her childhood and how it offered her a safe place to go during or after chemotherapy. Tapping into your memory may well help you to cope with feelings you're experiencing now. It might even offer insights which suggest ways forward.

1. A place from the past

(a) Choose a place either from your childhood or a later time that mattered to you. This could be a house where you once lived, a room in it or the garden, a school you attended, a park, a hideout, a field, a brook, a building or location where you did work you found satisfying or which you associate with someone you care about, etc. Begin by describing the place you've chosen. Don't worry if you can't remember many details. More may surface as you start writing. Include any feelings that come up. Move onto mentioning memories the place brings back. I made a short entry in my notebook on 31st May (Chapter Nine) about going out in a rowing boat. This was in Gourock on the Firth of Clyde where I spent most of my early childhood. Writing about this memory brought back the exuberance and sense of adventure I often felt as a child.

(b) If you would like to explore one of these memories further try writing in more detail about an incident, situation or person you connect with it, also how you felt then and your thoughts and feelings now as you look back. You might also find more material is unleashed if you use free association. Underline three sentences which strike you as key in the piece about a place in your past. Choose one of them and Flow-Write for a few minutes.

2. A person in your past

Choose a person who has had an influence on your life. This could be your partner, a parent, sibling, friend, teacher, someone you met briefly who changed your ideas, etc. Write about the person you've picked in any way you like. You might want to pinpoint one particular memory or to describe the person's character, appearance and way of life or you might want to focus on why you value her/him and how he/she has influenced you. In part my piece of writing 'The Cave' (5th April, Chapter Six) and the poem of the same title (2nd May, Chapter Eight) are about separating myself further from the influence of my dominating father. For Carole Satyamurti remembering lessons with her cello teacher was a way into writing a poem about fear. This is also from her sequence, 'Changing The Subject'.

Difficult Passages
by Carol Satyamurti

'You did not proper practise',
my cello teacher's sorrowful
mid-European vowels reproached me.
'Many times play through the piece
is not the proper practising
– you must repeat difficult passages
so when you make performance
there is not fear –you know
the music is inside your capacity.'
Her stabbing finger, moist gaze,
sought to plant the lesson in my soul.
I've practised pain for forty years
– all those Chinese burns;
the home-made dynamo we used
to test our tolerance for shocks;
hands wrapped round snowballs;
untreated corns – all pain practice.
Fine –if I can choose the repertoire.
But what if some day I'm required
to play a great pain concerto?
Will that be inside my capacity?

3. Positives in your past life

(a) Choose an activity that you have particularly enjoyed in your past life
either when you were a child or later. This might be roller-skating,
playing in a sandpit, going out for a meal, climbing, talking to friends
for half the night, making clothes, going to the pub, listening to music,

listening to stories a parent or other adult told you when you were a child, going to a disco, going for long walks, etc. Alternatively choose an exciting, satisfying or illuminating event: discovering you could read through a book, being given a pet, winning a swimming race, a secret game you played with friends, reading a book that made a strong impact, making a close friend, discovering you had an unexpected skill, being praised, etc. Describe the activity or incident, re-living it in as much detail as you can. Write about what you felt and include any other associations or thoughts which come into your mind. I wrote a piece in my notebook about going for walks on the South Downs when I was a teenager (see 8th August, Chapter Eleven).

(b) Make a list of three things you feel you've achieved in your life. These could be major achievements like getting the job or promotion you wanted, passing school exams, going to university, getting your first exhibition as an artist, overcoming a major difficulty or disadvantage, etc. Equally they could be apparently small scale achievements: passing your driving test after several attempts, learning to swim or some other skill, helping a friend or relative during a crisis, overcoming the fear of flying, standing up to a bully, learning to say 'no', learning deaf sign language, coming to terms with a situation you couldn't alter, etc. Choose one of these and write about it in as much detail as you like. Include how you felt about the achievement at the time and any thoughts or feelings you have about it now.

4. Key events in your life

Write down six key events or times of change in your life. These could be starting school, reaching puberty, leaving home, going to live in another country, starting your first job, a love affair, finding a partner, having a child, a promotion, etc. They might also include more difficult occurrences: a serious accident, separating from a partner, an unhappy relationship with a parent or child, the death of a parent or someone else close to you. Choose one of these events or changes to write about. Describe what happened and how you felt at the time.

How do you see it now? What have you gained from the experience? In the sonnet sequence, 'Knitting', Mary MacRae wrote during her illness she looks back at her childhood and how things changed for her as she grew up. She writes about how she

> ...made a vow
> not to join in, never to learn to sew,
> crochet or knit, use make-up, perm my hair,
> or wear high heels, (didn't keep that one);
> I found myself in books – Biggles, Dan Dare,
> or George of the Famous Five, not cry-baby Anne –
> nowhere else. But time was on my side,
> blue jeans and rock and roll arrived and then
> university, new life outside
> the Wendy House...

If you would like to explore your past further in writing you will find more ideas in *Writing for Self-Discovery*.

Playing with Words

Not long ago I was talking to two poet friends whose fathers had both been treated for cancer and we were soon discussing the fact that neither of these fathers could bring himself to use the word 'cancer'. Instead each referred to his illness with vague euphemisms like 'the old trouble'. It is understandable that the word still arouses terror even though during the past few decades, and especially the last one, more and more ways have been found to treat cancer effectively. Nevertheless it seems to me that fear and terror are much greater if they are *not* uttered. Dumping, as suggested in Letting Go in Lists, and Flow-Writing both offer ways of releasing frightening or difficult feelings. Another useful technique is to 'play' with them in words: make striking patterns with them, let off steam about them, wallow in them, guy them, fight back at them, laugh at them and in the process begin to explore them. Letting go and hitting back can be liberating and potent. Having a laugh is a wonderful way of reducing tension.

1. Patterning

(a) Choose an uncomfortable or difficult feeling you'd like to write about, maybe one you've been aware or half aware of but don't quite know how to tackle or one you feel the need to express more fully. This could be disgust, panic, anger, loneliness, restlessness, anxiety, envy, terror, powerlessness, being fed up, outrage, etc. Now write sentences about the feeling following (or mainly following) the same pattern: e.g. 'I'm fed up because...' or 'Anger is...' or some other very direct form which begins by pinpointing the feeling. As with Dumping start each sentence on a new line and put down whatever comes into your head without trying to think how accurate, important or logical it is.

It took me a while to recognize how angry I was about being ill. My first acknowledgement of the feeling was in an additional note to some Flow-Writing triggered by a painting. This was on 11th March (Chapter Five). Two months later, without any conscious decision, I found myself looking at my anger much more directly and writing a list mostly in a pattern (9th May, Chapter Eight). Here are a few lines from it:

> I'm angry if I drop something.
> I'm angry because I keep losing my glasses.
> I'm angry because the skin of my fingers is sore from chemo-
> therapy.
> I'm angry because my life's been interrupted.

(b) You might also like to try patterning round a feeling or mood you've found supportive or think you would find supportive, e.g. determination, hope, sympathy, acceptance, friendship, love, calm. Enjoy finding words which support this feeling.

(c) Now choose a loaded word or a word that is loaded for you. Make up a pattern and write a series of sentences or lines. Without planning to do so I found myself letting go in a pattern about the word 'cancer' very soon after I came home from hospital after my operation (14th February, Chapter Four):

Cancer the red scare word
the Gorgon fixing you with its eye word,
the big bad wolf in the wood word.

Other words might be 'operation', 'hospital', 'uncertainty', 'treat-ment', 'injection', 'realism', 'outcome', 'facing facts', 'Job's comforter', 'body', 'breast', 'hair', 'treatment', 'drug', etc. and there will probably be words which have a particular meaning for you at the moment.

(d) Now choose a sentence opening which relates to something that's been on your mind. This may have a connection with your illness or be some quite different matter. Early on before I had the operation I was worried about telling Erwin's cousin about my illness, feeling she might interfere and cast gloom about. In talking to friends who have had a serious illness or an upsetting bereavement I've discovered most of them have had some kind of problem in coping with a relative, friend or even an acquaintance who has rung up out of the blue and been very insensitive. One of the ways I coped with my anxiety about the insensitivity of others was to play with words. Both before the operation (2nd and 4th February, Chapter Two) and later on after I came home I made myself laugh out loud by thinking up more and more extravagant lines which began: 'I'm not going to tell her because...' It was a game but in the end I developed the lines into a poem (see 19th and 21st February, Chapter Four).

Here are some other possible openings: 'I'm in such a rage I could...', 'When the phone rings I'll...', 'I want to...', 'I'm so pissed off I could...', 'I don't want to...', 'I'm going to shout...', 'I wish I could...', 'Sod everything, I'll...', 'I'm going to...', etc. You may well prefer to think up your own opening. Have fun with it.

(e) You might also like to play with openings that spur you on or allow you to escape into a fantasy world, e.g. 'I'm going to jump on a plane and...', 'I'll climb a mountain and...', 'I'll go into the Ritz and...',

'When it's all over I'll…', etc. After my last chemotherapy session I felt I ought to have some sort of celebration. I wasn't up to 'going out on the town' but I thoroughly enjoyed making up lines beginning: 'When it's all over I'll…' and it was extremely satisfying to turn them into a poem (See 21st August, Chapter Eleven, 28th August, Chapter Twelve).

(f) Writing with a repeated word or phrase provides a strong pattern, a base form and you may well find yourself writing a poem even if you haven't written one before. In fact using a series of lines which follow the same pattern is a very good way into writing poetry. What begins as word play or letting off steam may be very potent as shaped expression of feelings and thoughts. One of the poems in Carole Satyamurti's sequence, 'Changing The Subject', is a series of short sentences following on from a title. Each begins with the word 'Because'. Apparently light, almost throw-away, the poem is sharp-edged and shows, without spelling it out, how having cancer has changed her vision of life. Here it is:

I Shall Paint My Nails Red
by Carole Satyamurti

Because a bit of colour is a public service.
Because I am proud of my hands.
Because it will remind me I'm a woman.
Because I will look like a survivor.
Because I can admire them in traffic jams.
Because my daughter will say ugh.
Because my lover will be surprised.
Because it is quicker than dyeing my hair.
Because it is a ten-minute moratorium.
Because it is reversible.

Try writing a poem or series of lines in a pattern which juxtaposes different moods or feelings. You could focus on opposing feelings/ideas in alternate lines or allow a second layer of feeling to filter through what appears to be the dominant mood.

2. Letting off steam

You may find that writing in a pattern is not sufficient. As the images build up you may want to let off steam in different ways about a feeling, situation or relationship or you may feel you need a different kind of space to explore an idea further. If this happens I suggest you try using a mix of letting off steam and Flow-Writing. Take the topic you want to write about. It can be something small that's bothering or irritating you or a feeling that seems to apply to all sorts of things: confusion, longing, fear, discomfort, depression, irritation, pretence, etc. It could also be a reaction to a major problem or experience. Write down the first sentence that comes into your head about your chosen topic and then, telling yourself this is your time for letting go, put down what comes into your head. On 9th May (Chapter Eight) after I'd done the 'angry' patterning, which I've mentioned in this section in Patterning (a), I found myself slapping words down on paper. It began with questions I didn't answer and then I simply let the anger rip, sometimes dropping into patterning. Here are a few lines:

> What does it feel like, this anger? What does it smell of? What does it sound like? It is bubbling in my body like a mob of prisoners. I want to throw it out, slap it like the sea on the shore. I shall shove it out like a bin of rubbish. I want to hit it into faces, wave it from steeples, dangle it in red flags...

It hadn't occurred to me that I could revel in being angry without bothering to attach the anger to something in particular. Letting off steam in this way gave me a marvellous sense of release and satisfaction. Using the material to write a poem gave me more scope to express my feelings and was great fun.

Image Explorations

Image explorations offer an opportunity to use your imagination to express feelings and travel your inner landscape without demanding that you analyse or explain. In some ways this technique is an extension of visualization. It is likely to take you away from your immediate preoccupations without necessarily losing connection with them. I found it had a remarkable effect when I tried out 'The Cave', an image exploration I'd devised for a writing course (5th April, Chapter Six). I am going to suggest four image explorations beginning with 'The Cave'. Try some of them and if you like this mode of writing you will find more ideas in *Writing for Self-Discovery*. I suggest you spend about ten minutes on each section of these explorations.

1. The cave

(a) Imagine you are by yourself in a cave. There is a little light but not much and it is very quiet. Picture the shape and size of the cave, its rock walls, ledges, crevices, whether there is any water or if you can see stalagmites or stalactites. Think about some of these things: the ground underfoot, the temperature, the dimness, the origin of what light there is, the smell. Write about what you can see, touch and smell, the atmosphere of the cave. Include your feelings and, if you want to, how you came to be in the cave.

(b)   You hear a sound or sounds which have a strong effect on you. Write about this.

(c)   You become aware of someone or something in the cave, maybe aware of more light. Find a way of developing the piece.

2. Crossing the bridge

(a)   You are on one side of a bridge. You want to cross it but the other side looks far away and the bridge presents dangers. It may be very narrow, or not a firm structure or it may have no sides. Looking down is frightening too. Picture the bridge, the far bank and your immediate surroundings as clearly as you can. Now describe what you can see, mentioning the dangers. Include why you want to cross and how you are feeling.

(b)   Steeling yourself, you step onto the bridge. You become aware of people on the other side. They are gesticulating and calling out to you. Write about this and how it affects you.

(c)   Write about what happens next.

3. Climbing a mountain

(a)   You are by yourself climbing a mountain. You have already come a long way. There are rocks, ravines and steep slopes below you but the top of the mountain still seems far off. You feel very alone. Describe what you can see, mention the weather, what provisions you have and how you are feeling.

(b) You come across someone resting on a boulder. You talk to this person and at first are bothered, worried, or upset by what he/she is saying. Gradually you gain a different impression. Write about this encounter.

(c) Develop the piece.

4. The safe place

(a) You are in a strange street, alley, corridor, passage or some other location where you feel afraid. It may be you are frightened of someone or something specific or your fear may be undefined. You are searching for a place where you will be safe. Write about this.

(b) You come upon a room, cubby-hole, niche, quiet garden, bed or other place which offers the refuge you seek. Describe going into it and how it affects you.

(c) The safe place reminds you of another time when you felt safe or maybe of people who gave you comfort and security in the past, or you may be experiencing a feeling of safety that you've not found before. Write about your associations and feelings.

Try making up your own image explorations. Give your imagination free reign and it will lead you to what you want to write about. Here is a list of features which might be useful for reference: steps, flying, eggs, a tree, a blindfold, the sea, a tower, a train, a telephone, a gate, a wall, a door, an elephant, a key, a see-saw.

Taking an Overview

As time goes on after you've recuperated from an operation or as you are recovering from chemotherapy and/or radiotherapy, you may find it helpful to take stock of what has happened to you and how it has changed your life. Talking about your illness to understanding friends and other people who've had cancer or to a counsellor is likely to be very supportive. Writing can also be a therapeutic and illuminating way of recording and assimilating the experience you've been through, a way to explore your new perspective.

1. Negatives and positives

As a first step I suggest you begin by making a list of losses and then a list of gains. Losses might include: loss of a part of your body – maybe a part of your body connected with sexuality; loss of immunity or sensation in one area of your body; loss of fertility, of hair, of time from your life, of energy; giving up a job; loss of time with children; loss of security, of confidence; a sense of powerlessness, etc. Gains might include: new understanding and insights; a new and deeper appreciation of life; a removal from strains at work or elsewhere; new friends; time for yourself at home to read, to write, to meditate, watch birds in the garden. They might also include: a new determination; a decision to change your job; to move to a different environment; to commit yourself to creative work or a new activity or to study something you've always intended to but never made time for.

As a second step read through the two lists and write a continuous piece or notebook entry which sets the negatives and positives side by side. This will give you an overview of your experience of cancer.

When artist, Anna Adams, had breast cancer in the 1960s, she had two small sons and methods of treatment were nothing like as advanced as they are now. After her illness she started writing poetry much more urgently because she had a new sense of life's shortness. Her first collection was published in 1979. She is now a well-known poet and has had several more collections published including *Green Resistance*, her new and selected poems.

2. Exploring issues

It is very possible that there is an item (or items) on one of your lists which is a central issue for you, something you want to explore in depth in order to release yourself from it, absorb it, understand it better or come to terms with it. Towards the end of her sequence, 'Changing The Subject', Carole Satyamurti found different ways of contemplating the fear of dying which, of course, becomes much more real if one has cancer, even if the prognosis is very good. Three of these poems are included in Writing Ideas: 'Choosing the Furniture' (Visualizations), 'Difficult Passages' (Writing About Memories), 'I Shall Paint My Nails Red' (Playing with Words).

If you've had a mastectomy losing a breast is likely to be a key issue. You have already seen that I have written about this in many different ways in my notebook and in poems. The night before her mastectomy Alicia Stubbersfield wrote a short poem in her notebook:

Goodbye to my left breast
by Alicia Stubbersfield

Warm, soft, a small handful,
big nipple that comforted Joe,
the side next to my heart
where he slept easier.
One freckle on the aureola.
Curved upwards, full underneath,
I can't hold a pencil there,
struggled to place you for the mammogram.
Men have loved you, touched you naked
or through layers of clothes.
No more –

I shall be an Amazon
single-breasted warrior,
paddling in crocodile waters
towards a strange dappled light
and in the distance the sound
of drums.

Later Alicia wrote a notebook entry which commented sharply on the
difficulty of dealing with the practical reality of only having one
breast:

> We all went to Cardiff which felt quite odd really. I wore my
> black linen trousers and black shirt with a strategically placed
> scarf. Fine. The lingerie department in Howells was full of
> brightly coloured padded bras like sweets and 'Breast Aware-
> ness Month' pink ribbons. I felt like Tom Robinson in the sev-
> enties with an auditorium of straight people singing along to

Glad to be Gay. Not one sign of the reality of a mastectomy. I asked a girl for suitable bras and she just said they didn't have any. I bought a little soft Calvin Klein top and shorts. Very tired by the end but I'd managed.

I am going to suggest some ways of writing about central subjects. You may know at once how you want to tackle your issue in which case, of course, go ahead.

(a) If you're not quite sure what you want to focus on or if you're aware of a welter of feelings and thoughts I suggest you begin with a mixture of Dumping and Flow-Writing. I've already described Dumping in Letting Go in Lists. I think this is a very potent and indicative method. Simply note down anything and everything that occurs to you about the subjects on your mind. Write in shortish sentences starting each one on a new line and keep to a sentence pattern as much as you can. When you've finished the list read it through and underline any sentence or thought which you would like to write about in more detail. Now take one of the underlined sentences or phrases. Write it down and continue with Flow-Writing – writing whatever comes into your head – for about six minutes, longer if you want to. Look at your Flow-Writing and underline anything which interests you. You may now have the material to write a continuous piece about your burning issue or you may want to collect more material first by doing a second session of Flow-Writing using one of your underlined sentences.

(b) If you're clear about the subject you want to explore further but don't know how to get into it, write down the first sentence about it which comes into your head and go straight into Flow-Writing for several minutes. Even if you've already done Flow-Writing round this topic before it will be helpful to do it again. Underline what interests you in your Flow-Writing. This is likely to tell you what you want to focus on in a continuous piece of writing.

(c) If the subject you're exploring or want to explore is very painful you might find it helpful to start by writing a visualization round it. You could adapt visualization (d) in the third section of Visualizations which focuses on healing. Imagine putting the details which distress you into a box or chest but instead of shutting it away out of sight, picture yourself putting the partly open box somewhere where you can view it safely – perhaps on the other side of a double-glazed window. Alternatively you could imagine giving the box to someone or more than one person who will take charge of it and be supportive as you look at its contents together. Or you may come up with quite a different visualization which will help you approach the issue you want to write about.

(d) You might find it helpful to write a straight notebook piece in which you look at your issue from different angles and examine it in some detail. If it's appropriate include ways in which you can support yourself or get support in dealing with it. In my entries for 2nd October (Chapter Twelve) and 8th November (Chapter Thirteen) I looked at the difficulties I was having in coping with the recovery period.

Taking Your Writing Further

You may find you would like to give more shape to some of your pieces of raw writing or journal entries or that there is material you would like to explore in much more depth. There might be subjects you would like to write about which you've not yet tackled. Mary MacRae felt having breast cancer was a major turning point in her life. She wrote in her notebook:

> A time to understand what's happened, how it's changed me
> and what different lines it draws in the sand.

Because of her illness she had to give up a responsible teaching post which she loved. However, one of the positive things that came out of this was that at last she could find the time she badly wanted for writing poetry.

Soon after her mastectomy Mary had a dream about knitting the strands of her life together. This was the trigger for 'Knitting', a sequence of fifteen sonnets in which images of 'clicking the steel needles', unravelling and knitting up recur as she looks over her life, in particular at her links with her mother and her daughter, and also her experience of cancer. The sequence opens with a paradox: 'Never did

learn to knit.' The poems were written while she was undergoing chemotherapy and later they were published in the journal *Scintilla*. In the
third sonnet she draws on her memory of the dream to describe
waking up from her operation, how her body feels and her relief that
the cancerous breast has been removed. It ends with images which
show her uncertainty of the way ahead. I think the poem carries a
strong sense of rebirth. Here it is:

> I dream of holding different coloured strands,
> cat's cradle hammock, swinging in the shade,
> then wake. I'm cold, alone, can't move, tight band
> around my chest, arm bent to touch right side.
> Flat. Good. Exhale. Yes, I'm sure. It's gone.
> Half a child again, I want to keep
> my secret safe. Now I'm Amazon
> though, for the moment, baby-swaddled. Sleep.
> My bow arm's numb. I jettison my arrows
> but something sharp's still sticking into me
> like a row of pins along my front, narrow
> line of stuck zip fastener. Gingerly,
> I tug. Zip or unzip? Which way now? –
> clicking the steel needles to find out how?

You may feel you would like to write about your illness in the context
of the rest of your life or feel like exploring different areas of your life.
There are other possibilities for taking your writing further. It could be
that you would like to write an article for a magazine or newspaper
about an aspect of your illness. Alicia Stubbersfield's note about her
visit to a department store to try and buy a suitable bra in 'Breast
Awareness Month' could have been expanded into an article drawing
attention to the pointlessness of paying lip service to ideas and needs.
Even in her note the implications of her criticism go far. The same

material could also have provided the starting point for a biting short story. An illuminating or humorous incident about how you coped with a difficult situation might be developed into an article which would be supportive to other people.

If you have written a poem or poems during your illness you may have found that you enjoyed searching out words and shaping them, feel you would like to pinpoint more moments, feelings, insights in poems. You might want to write poems on themes which are not connected with illness. Perhaps you have all kinds of ideas you would like to explore in prose, possibly in fiction.

If you have been keeping a diary or notebook maybe you would find it valuable to continue with it after the main period of your illness is over. Whether a journal is written up frequently or at irregular intervals this form of writing, which can be so supportive and illuminating in a time of stress or change, is potent at any time. In *44½ Choices you can make if you have cancer* Vicki Golding, who already kept a journal before she had cancer, explains why it was so important to her:

> Writing a journal had the same effect as crying – I was able to get out what I was feeling in a way that I couldn't do with anyone I know. It was also very useful to look back. I felt compelled to write, at first only for myself, then later to share with others.

One of her co-writers, Jo Wright, also turned to writing for support when she was undergoing treatment for cancer:

> Although I've never kept a diary I felt a strong desire to write down my thoughts. It helped me straighten out in my mind how I was feeling. At first when I was writing everything seemed to be a jumble but by writing it down my thoughts seemed to make more sense.

A few days after her mastectomy Alicia Stubbersfield wrote this piece in her notebook:

> Today I can't get comfortable. The drain stings and drags. I talk to too many people on the phone and feel sick. The first

Tamoxifen – the marker. This defines me now at the optician, dentist, everywhere.

I'm weeping today – for myself because I'm afraid of dying. I read about Ruth Picardie and shouldn't have. I get up for dinner. I could lie in bed drowning in tears for ever and that won't do. My night was so bad it extended into the day. Manic images of the hospital.

Oddly I feel released from my mother at last – this is my body, different from hers though the disease is the same, my scar embroidered by Mr. Jones. And my own fight which I can do – not under her shadow.

In a short space Alicia lets out different feelings of distress, fear and disorientation and the remarkable last paragraph pinpoints an insight and marks a change of mood to determination.

Whether you decide to keep a journal or to try other kinds of writing, whether you write occasionally or often, whether what you write is for yourself or to share with others, I hope you will find, as I did, that writing is a way to make sense of the journey through illness, a way to create something meaningful out of an extreme experience.

Other Books by Myra Schneider

Poetry collections

Fistful of Yellow Hope. Littlewood Press (1984) Hebden Bridge, Yorkshire.

Cat Therapy. Littlewood Press (1986; reprinted 1989) Todmordon, Lancashire.

Cathedral of Birds. Littlewood/Giant Steps (1988) Todmordon, Lancashire.

Opening The Ice (with Ann Dancy). Smith/Doorstop (1990) Huddersfield, Yorkshire.

Crossing Point. Littlewood Press (1991) Todmordon, Lancashire.

Exits. Enitharmon (1994) London.

The Panic Bird. Enitharmon (1998) London.

Insisting on Yellow: New and Selected Poems. Enitharmon (2000) London.

Forthcoming: *Multiplying The Moon.* Enitharmon (2004) London.

Fiction for children and teenagers

Marigold's Monster. Heinemann (1976) London.

If Only I Could Walk. Heinemann (1977) London.

Will The Real Pete Roberts Stand Up? Heinemann (1978) London.

Non-fiction

Writing for Self-Discovery (with John Killick). Vega, Chrysalis Books (2002) London. (Element 1998; Barnes & Noble USA1999)

Anthologies edited

Parents (co-edited with Dilys Wood). An anthology of poems by women writers about their parents. Enitharmon (2000) London.

Making Worlds (co-edited with Gladys Mary Coles and Dilys Wood). A major anthology of poetry by contemporary women poets. Headland (2003) West Kirby, Mersyside.

Bibliography

Adams, Anna (1996) *Green Resistance: New and Selected Poems.* London: Enitharmon.

Atkinson, Kate (1996) *Behind the Scenes at the Museum.* London: Black Swan.

Clifton, Lucille (1999) *The Terrible Stories.* USA: Slow Dancer Press.

Cluysenaar, Anne (1997) *Timeslips.* Manchester: Carcanet.

Dainow, Sheila, Golding, Vicki and Wright, Jo (2001) *44½ Choices You Can Make if You Have Cancer.* Dublin: Gill & Macmillan.

Fanthorpe, U.A. (2000) *Consequences.* Calstock, Cornwall: Peterloo Poets.

Feinstein, Elaine (2000) *Gold.* Manchester: Carcanet.

Hesketh, Phoebe (1994) *The Leave Train: New and Selected Poems.* London: Enitharmon.

Khalvati, Mimi (1997) *Entries on Light.* Manchester: Carcanet.

Khalvati, Mimi (2000) *Selected Poems.* Manchester: Carcanet.

Khalvati, Mimi (2002) 'Writing Letters' and 'Writing Home.' In *The Chine.* Manchester: Carcanet.

Killick, John (1996) *Windhorse.* Ware: Rockingham Press (11 Musley Lane, Ware, Herts SG12 7EN).

Killick, John (1997) 'You Are Words: Dementia Poems.' *The Journal of Dementia Care.* London: Hawker Publications Ltd. (13 Park House, 140 Battersea Park Road, London SW11 4NB).

Killick, John (2000) 'Openings: Dementia Poems and Photographs.' *The Journal of Dementia Care.* London: Hawker Publications.

Lindop, Grevel (1996) *The Path and The Path and The Palace.* London: Temenos Academy (14 Gloucester Gate, London, NW1 4HG).

Lindop, Grevel (2000) 'Summer pudding.' In *Selected Poems.* Manchester: Carcanet.

Livingstone, Dinah (2000) *The Poetry of Earth.* London: Katabasis (10 St. Martin's Close, London NW1 OHR).

MacRae, Mary (2000) 'Knitting.' In *Scintilla*. Gwent: Usk Valley Vaughan Association.

MacRae, Mary (1999) 'Appointment.' In *Magma*. London: Magma.

Murray, Les (1991) *Collected Poems*. Manchester: Carcanet.

Rospigliosi, Veronica (1999) *Reckitt's Blue*. London: Hearing Eye Press (Box 1, 99 Torriano Avenue, London NW5 2RX).

Rowbotham, Colin (2002) *Lost Connections: New and Selected Poems*. London: Arnos Press (34 Willes Road, London NW5 3DS).

Sacks, Oliver (1995) *An Anthropologist on Mars*. London: Picador.

Satyamurti, Carole (2000) 'Changing the subject.' In *Selected Poems*. Highgrren, Tarset, Northumberland: Bloodaxe. Oxford University Press, 1998.

Schneider, Myra (2000) *Insisting on Yellow: New and Selected Poems*. London: Enitharmon.

Schneider, Myra (2000) *The Panic Bird*. London: Enitharmon.

Schneider, Myra and Killick, John (2002) *Writing for Self-Discovery*. London: Vega, Chrysalis Books.

Stevenson, Anne (1996) 'A Tunnel of Summers.' In *Collected Poems 1955–1995*. Oxford: Oxford University Press.

Stevenson, Anne (2000) 'Arioso Dolente.' In *Granny Scarecrow* (Bloodaxe) and *Parents: An Anthology by Women Writers* (London: Enitharmon).

van de Molen, Beverley (2003) *Taking Control of Cancer*. London: Class Publishing.

Vaughan, Henry (1996) *The Complete Poems*. Edited by Alan Rudrum. London: Penguin.

Williams, C.K. (1996) 'Train', 'Ice' and 'Invisible Mending.' *Repair*. Highgreen, Tarset, Northumberland: Bloodaxe.

Williams, C.K. (1997) *The Vigil*. Highgreen, Tarset, Northumberland: Bloodaxe.

Literary journals and poetry magazines

Magma
43 Keslake Road
London NW6 6DH
email: magmapoems@aol.com

The North
The Poetry Business
The Studio
Byram Arcade
Westgate
Huddersfield HD1 1ND
email: edit@poetrybusiness.co.uk

Scintilla (an annual publication of the Usk Valley Vaughan Association)
Little Wentwood Farm
Llantrisant
Usk
Gwent NP15 1ND.
email: anne.cluysenaar@virgin.net

Quadrant
437 Darling Street
Balmain
NSW 2041
Australia
email: quadrantmonthly@ozmail.com.au

Useful Addresses

Writing

Lapidus
Organization promoting the use of the literary arts in personal development. Its members are therapists, teachers, poets and others who believe in the value of personal writing. It operates as a network, has a newsletter and magazine and conferences. Regional groups hold meetings.

Address: BM Lapidus, London WC1N 3XX
Website: www.lapidus.org.uk
email: Pam_Thorne@arian.demon.co.uk

The Poetry Library
A comprehensive collection of twentieth century and contemporary poetry with sections for reference and lending. Membership is free. Large selection of contemporary poetry magazines, poetry on cassette, information about poetry courses, workshops, groups, poetry festivals, venues, competitions; offers information worldwide about poetry organizations.

Telephone: 020 7921 0943/0664
Address: Level Five, The Royal Festival Hall, London SE1 8XX
Opening Times: 11a.m.–8p.m. Tuesday–Sunday, closed Monday except for telephone enquiries
Website: www.poetrylibrary.org.uk
email: info@poetrylibrary.org.uk

The Poetry School
Offers courses in reading and writing poetry, workshops, small group seminars, lectures, special events and tutorials including postal tutorials. Mainly based in London but some events and seminars outside London. People from other parts of the country travel to London to attend workshops, lectures and special events.

Telephone: 020 8223 0401 (Administrator: Jacqueline Gabbitas)
Address: 1a Jewel Road, Walthamstow, London E17 4QU
Website: www.poetryschool.com
E-mail: programme@poetryschool.com

Second Light
Network for women poets, aged around 40 and upwards, who are serious
about developing their work. Associate membership for younger poets. Aims
to develop members' work and promote poetry by women. Newsletter,
readings, workshops, annual conference in Leicestershire, annual poetry
competition, produces anthologies of women's poetry in co-operation with
key publishers.

Address: Dilys Wood (Co-ordinator), 9 Greendale Close, London SE22 8TG
Website: www.esch.dircon.co.uk (page about Second Light from Myra
Schneider's website)
email: dilyswood@tiscali.co.uk

Note
Myra Schneider runs or co-runs with John Killick occasional one-off
workshops which focus on personal writing and is sometimes available to
run workshops.
Address: 130 Morton Way, Southgate, London N14 7AL
Website: www.esch.dircon.co.uk
email: myra.sch@ukonline.co.uk

United States

National Association of Poetry Therapy
Membership association for psychotherapists, social workers, poets, journal
keepers, teachers, students, doctors, nurses and others who believe that words
and all forms of literature can be used to help heal individuals and bring
together communities.

Telephone: Toll-free within US on 1 866 844 NAPT or (001)954 499 4333
Address: 12950 NW 5th Street, Pembroke Pines, Florida 33028–3102
Website: www.poetrytherapy.org
email: info@poetrytherapy.org

General

BACUP
Umbrella cancer organization which helps people with cancer, their families and friends live with cancer. Specialist cancer nurses provide information, emotional support and practical advice by telephone, letter and email. Free publications available and they also offer free one-to-one counselling.

Freephone, Cancer Information Service. 0808 800 1234 (Monday–Friday 9a.m.–7p.m.)
Address: 3 Bath Place, Rivington Street, London EC2A 3JR
Website: www.cancerbacup.org.uk

Breast Cancer Care
The leading provider of breast cancer information across the UK and committed to offering practical and emotional support to everyone affected by breast cancer. Its services, all free, include a helpline staffed by specialist nurses and trained volunteers many of whom have had personal experience of breast cancer, also publications and a newsletter.

Freephone Helpline: 0808 800 6000 (Monday–Friday 10a.m.-5p.m., Saturday 10a.m.–2p.m.) textphone 0808 800 6001
Address: Kiln House, 210 New Kings Road, London SW6 4NZ
Website: www.breastcancercare.org.uk
email: info@breastcancer.org.uk

The British Association for Counselling and Psychotherapy
Umbrella membership body for counselling and psychotherapy. Provides information on counselling services locally.

Telephone: 0870 443 5252
Address: 1 Regent Place, Rugby, Warwickshire CV21 2PJ
Website: www.bac.co.uk
email: bac@bac.co.uk

The Haven Trust
A national charity offering information, advice and complementary therapies (including creative writing) free of charge, for anyone affected by breast cancer. Based in Fulham. A new centre due to open in 2003 in Hereford.

Helpline: 0870 727 2273
Address: Effie Road, Fulham, London SW6 1TB
Website: www.thehaventrust.org.uk
email: info@thehaventrust.org.uk

The Helen Rollason Cancer Care Centre Appeal
This charity is in the process of setting up a nationwide network of centres
to provide information, complementary treatments and support to people
diagnosed with cancer.

Telephone: 0124 551 3350
Address: Room 2, Wood House, St John's Hospital, Wood Street,
Chelmsford, Essex CM2 9BB
Website: www.healcancercharity.org.uk
email: helenrollason.appeal@virgin.net

Macmillan Cancerline
Provides emotional support and information on all aspects of cancer to
people with cancer, family, friends and professionals working with them.
Supports self-help groups throughout Britain. Offers free publications and
audiotapes in several languages.

Freephone Helpline: 0808 808 2020 (Monday–Friday 9a.m.–6p.m.)
Address: Cancerlink, 89 Albert Embankment, London SE1 7UQ
Website: www.cancerlink.org

Spectrum
Humanistic psychotherapy practice with trained therapists working
throughout the country.

Telephone: 020 8341 2277
Address: 7 Endymion Road, Finsbury Park, London N4 1EE
Website: www.spectrumtherapy.co.uk

The UK Council for Psychotherapy (UKCP)
Professional organization with national register from which members of the
public can identify therapists local to them.

Telephone: 020 7436 3002
Address: 167–169 Great Portland Street, London W1W 5PF
Website: www.psychotherapy.org.uk

Cassette: Relaxation and Self-Healing

This tape includes a relaxation exercise with breathing awareness and meditation exercises which help ground, relax and revitalize the listener. Can be ordered direct. Send a cheque payable for £7.70 to 'Kate Williams MacKenzie'. Orders from outside the UK will be accepted (also for £7.70) provided payment is made in pounds sterling. (Please check current price before ordering.)

Address: Kate Williams MacKenzie, Forest Lodge, Inverness IV2 7HT
Website: www.katewilliamsmackenzie.com
email: katewilliamsworkingwithpeople@btinternet.com

United States

Cancer Care Inc.
National non-profit making organization whose main aim is to offer professional help to people with all cancers and their careers through continuing education, information, referral and direct financial assistance. Telephone counselling offered.

Telephone: (001) 800 813 4673 (toll free in the US)
Address: 275 7th Avenue, NY 10001, New York, USA
Website: www.cancercare.org
email: info@cancercare.org

American Cancer Society
This organization offers detailed information about cancer and about resources in different areas. It also offers information and help by phone and they can be emailed directly from their website.

Telephone: (001) 800 227 2345 (toll free in the US)
Address: National Home Office, 1599 Clifton Road, NE Atlanta, GA 30329-4251, USA
Website: www.cancer.org

Index